Osteoporosis

ALSO BY WILLIAM N. TAYLOR, M.D.

Macho Medicine:
A History of the Anabolic Steroid Epidemic
(McFarland, 1991)

Hormonal Manipulation:
A New Era of Monstrous Athletes
(McFarland, 1985)

Anabolic Steroids and the Athlete
(McFarland, 1982)

Marathon Running:
A Medical Science Handbook
(McFarland, 1982)

Osteoporosis

Medical Blunders and Treatment Strategies

WILLIAM N. TAYLOR, M.D.

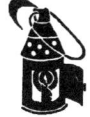

McFarland & Company, Inc., Publishers
Jefferson, North Carolina, and London

Cover illustration: The posturing of the same woman prior to menopause, during the perimenopause and at postmenopause. Notice the significant reduction in stature and anterior curving of the spine due to anterior compression fractures in the postmenopausal drawing. Notice also that the rib cage actually begins to touch the pelvis and that the abdominal cavity protrudes forward in the postmenopausal drawing. Due to the compression of the entire truncal region, lung capacity is greatly reduced in the postmenopausal case.

Advisory: This book is not intended as a medical manual. Neither the publisher nor the author is responsible for health consequences that may result from any course of treatment described herein. Anyone seeking diagnosis of a possible medical condition, or a prescription for treatment, should see a physician for evaluation.

British Library Cataloguing-in-Publication data are available

Library of Congress Cataloguing-in-Publication Data

Taylor, William N.
    Osteoporosis : medical blunders and treatment strategies / William N. Taylor, M.D.
      p. cm.
    Includes bibliographical references and index.
    ISBN 0-7864-0229-6 (sewn softcover : 55# alk. paper) ∞
    1. Osteoporosis. I. Title.
      [DNLM: 1. Osteoporosis — diagnosis. 2. Osteoporosis — prevention & control.   WE 250 T247o 1996]
RC931.073T39   1996
616.7'16 — dc20
DNLM/DLC
for Library of Congress   96-21046
                                                                              CIP

©1996 William N. Taylor. All rights reserved

No part of this book, specifically including the index, may be reproduced or transmitted in any form or by any means, electronic or mechanical, including photocopying or recording, or by any information storage and retrieval system, without permission in writing from the publisher.

Manufactured in the United States of America

McFarland & Company, Inc., Publishers
  Box 611, Jefferson, North Carolina 28640

This book is dedicated to
Earline Merritt Taylor, my mother,
for her continual inspiration
and for her acceptances
of both my successes and failures.
Her love for me has never wavered.

Acknowledgments

I would like to salute the memory of Robert B. Greenblatt, M.D., obstetrician and endocrinologist, for his pioneering work and his courageous determination never to let the medical truth in this area of medicine die. Fortunately, I was privileged to be able to thank him in person prior to his death.

For fifty years the medical establishment essentially rebuffed and ignored his important research and insightful concepts regarding the successful medical management of menopausal and postmenopausal issues. His major emphasis was on attempting to mimic the normal production of the ovarian sex steroids for his menopausal and postmenopausal patients. He pioneered the replacement of estrogen and androgen combinations, and he was not only correct in these areas, but was admirably persistent in disseminating his results over the decades. He was one of a few medical pioneers who was finally recognized, albeit only to a minimal degree, after his death. Unfortunately, encumbered by its collective egos, the medical profession sometimes treats its most intelligent pioneers in similar fashion.

Dr. Greenblatt's publications have taught me more about the sex steroids in women than any single one of my medical professors ever

Acknowledgments

did. Although I was never fortunate enough to take a course from Dr. Greenblatt, his medical publications provided me with invaluable medical facts regarding the physiology of the sex steroids. All I had to do was to take the time to read them, and the same opportunity still exists for every single one of my medical colleagues as well.

The book that follows is my contribution to his legacy and my tribute to his genius. It is my attempt to help millions of American women and men who suffer from the disease called osteoporosis — sometimes without knowing it, and in the vast majority of cases, completely unnecessarily.

Table of Contents

Acknowledgments — vii
Preface — 1
Introduction — 5

1: Building Blocks of the Epidemic — 13
2: The Period of Sex Steroid Experimentation — 19
3: The Period of False Dogma — 43
4: The Proper Diagnosis, Treatment, Reversal and Cure of Osteoporosis — 47
5: Alarming Physician Attitudes — 69
6: Contemporary Questions and Answers — 79

Afterword — 93
Bibliography — 95
About the Author — 101
Index — 103

Preface

Osteoporosis is an epidemic in the United States — an epidemic of major importance with serious multifaceted consequences. I have been calling the national osteoporosis predicament an epidemic for years, based on compelling data that support this designation. Consider the following statistics, some of which are compiled by the National Osteoporosis Foundation:

- More than 50 percent of white American women over the age of 45 years already have some degree of osteoporosis;
- More than 85 percent of white American women over the age of 70 years have osteoporosis;
- More than 1.2 million bone fractures annually are due to osteoporosis;
- More than $12 billion annually are spent treating the ill-health consequences of osteoporosis, with some estimates ranging in excess of $30 billion annually;
- More than 200,000 women are expected to sustain a debilitating hip fracture due to osteoporosis in 1996;
- One in five women who sustain a hip fracture and who do

Preface

not die as an immediate result will require long-term nursing home care and suffer a drastic decline in the quality of life, such as crippling pain, lasting disability, forced retirement and permanent disfigurement;

• One out of two women, following menopause, will sustain an osteoporosis-related hip fracture; and

• A woman's risk of an osteoporosis-related hip fracture is equal to her *combined* risk of developing breast, uterine or ovarian cancer.

Osteoporosis is perhaps the most common chronic disease in white American women currently. Can you think of a disease process, other than death, that affects more than 85 percent of all white women over the age of 70 years? I cannot. Not even heart disease is that prevalent. For most white women, osteoporosis is an eventual fact of life — but it is also preventable, treatable and, in some cases, curable.

The keys for the prevention, reversal and even cure for this frightening disease, as you will discover later in this book, are relatively simple and inexpensive. But the appropriate therapy depends on individualizing the proper replacement of the three classes of sex steroids that the ovaries made naturally when the woman was younger.

I wonder why people act as if they don't care about the only body which they will ever have. It is obvious to me, as a concerned physician who has practiced for many years, that many people do not. I am hoping that this phenomenon is not due to ignorance, or apathy, or worse, some combination of both. The combination of ignorance and apathy is very hard to overcome.

It makes me angry that most Americans seem to be too lazy to learn about one of the largest medical epidemics the world has ever seen, one which will eventually affect most of us directly or indirectly. Some of this anger is due to the fact that it is, more and more, the insurance companies who are practicing medicine without a medical license. And specifically with osteoporosis, some of this anger is provoked by some of the recalcitrant older women who either go against good medical advice or choose to faithfully follow the advice of physi-

Preface

cians who have not gotten out from under the misinformation disseminated years ago.

Is there anyone alive today who actually believes that significant shrinking in adult height is a normal phenomenon of aging? You bet there is; just ask any elderly woman. Her medical doctor or chiropractor probably told her so, if she was even concerned enough to ask. Somehow, it has been rationalized that losing several inches in adult height is normal, and older women have accepted this notion. How many people, either medical professionals or laypersons, think that osteoporosis is a normal aging process that has no cure or solution? What is this opinion based on, the mere fact that it has never been reversed or cured before?

Tax dollars are being spent at a record pace, seemingly ignoring new, innovative, effective, and more cost-efficient medical treatments for diseases which can be prevented or detected very early. Instead of supporting these new preventative measures, precious health care dollars are used to pay for the consequences of osteoporosis just because of the seeming complacency of physicians and patients alike. The osteoporosis epidemic leaches calcium from our skeletons and dollars from our wallets each and every day. There is a solution and in some cases a cure. We can defeat this disease and the suffering it causes if we work together and if we care. Medical ignorance and societal apathy have too high a price tag, physically and financially, for us to accept.

Introduction

Osteoporosis may be defined as a reduction in bone mass per unit volume of bone such that bone fractures may occur as a result of minimal or no trauma. This reduction in bone mass is mostly the loss of calcium and associated matrix structure, which results in the loss of structural integrity and strength of bones. Simply put, osteoporosis means porous and brittle bones.

This loss of calcium and other minerals, also known as bone mineral density, can now be identified safely, accurately, longitudinally, and early in the course of the disease process. Early diagnosis of the disease process is important for early intervention and treatment programs.

Osteoporosis is *not* a normal aging process. Most osteoporosis begins when a normal aging process occurs, namely the diminished production of sex steroids. It occurs whenever the normal bone cell equilibrium is upset for an extended period of time, and it can occur in men.

Sex steroid hormones play major roles in maintaining the normal bone cell equilibrium, the appropriate sex steroid therapy may prevent, reverse and perhaps cure most cases of osteoporosis through

Introduction

these steroids' effects on the various types of bone cells involved with this equilibrium process. Other hormones and minerals are involved with this equilibrium process, but the major factors are the various types of sex steroids. Therefore, the keys to understanding the osteoporosis process are linked to understanding the basic sex steroid biochemistry as it relates to bone cells, which will be discussed later in this book.

Osteoporosis is perhaps the most common chronic disease among American white women today, and it is the most common metabolic bone disease in the Western World. By far the most prevalent and most important type is postmenopausal osteoporosis, which will correspondingly receive the most emphasis in this book.

There are many causes of osteoporosis, but the postmenopausal variety results from a diminished or discontinued production of certain sex steroids following either the natural "change of life" or the surgical removal of both of a woman's ovaries prior to menopause. Osteoporosis will affect most white women by the end of their lives.

Despite a slowly increasing awareness of the importance of osteoporosis, many women do not know that they may have it or that it may be preventable, reversible or even curable. There are numerous risk factors which have been associated with the eventual development of osteoporosis, but the disease is so common among premenopausal and postmenopausal white women that the need for risk factor assessment is essentially obviated. (It is vastly less common, though not unknown, among black women, who in general attain significantly higher peak bone mineral densities during adolescence and the early adult years and maintain higher levels throughout life. The reasons for this difference are not known.)

National screening of white women above the age of 35 years is at least as important as routine screening of women for all types of cancers combined. Why? Simply put, osteoporosis is more common than all cancers in women combined, and there are definitive detection and treatment modalities available.

Traditionally, there has been some confusion about the medical terms *osteoporosis* and *osteopenia*. Osteopenia has been described as

Introduction

the loss of bone mineral density without any bone fractures occurring yet. In truth, postmenopausal osteopenia and osteoporosis are both exactly the same process, and the two terms merely refer to different parts of the same disease continuum.

Because of the influence and financial impact of some health insurance carriers and the government, which have balked at "covering" this disease condition, some arbitrary lines have been drawn between osteopenia and osteoporosis. Within this text, however, these terms will be considered synonymous.

The American public needs to become educated about and serious about osteoporosis. Imagine that a woman's bones can become so weak and brittle that, just by bearing the weight of standing up, one of her hips may fracture.

For many women, just the weight of the head can begin to crush the vertebrae in the neck and cause chronic pain. Eventually, the weight of the head may crush enough of the neck vertebrae to give rise to the classic rounded upper back and neck, or "dowager's hump."

I have seen many women leaving doctors' offices with undiagnosed and untreated osteoporosis. How can this be? Don't these physicians know or care what will be in store for their women patients? Some of the reason that physicians fail to pay osteoporosis its due may be due to the policies of some health insurance carriers. Traditionally, the health insurance carriers have refused to cover the expense of the definitive scans which can detect osteoporosis, especially in its earliest stages.

In other words, most of our health insurance carriers have adopted the stance of waiting until a woman suffers a hip fracture before her insurance policy kicks in to cover the diagnostic testing for osteoporosis. Of course, by that point, it may be too late. One in five women will die within the six months following an osteoporosis-related hip fracture or its complications, and many of the ones who survive this event will become nursing home patients. Incredibly, as of this writing, the largest military health insurance carrier will not cover the only definitive, accurate and safe method of detecting osteoporosis at any stage of the disease.

Introduction

All of this makes one wonder what ever happened to concern for the patient or to preventive medicine. Many physicians, politicians, and the health insurers talk about preventive medicine, but for the most part, their support for it is mere lip service. The net result is that osteoporosis and its related problems — which may include the fracture of any bone, and the subsequent pain, disfigurement, and disability resulting from these fractures — are costing American taxpayers over $30 billion annually. The actual costs, however, are surely impossible to measure or to predict now or in the future.

Most certainly, the estimates and actual health care expenditures spent fighting this crippling disease will skyrocket as the American lifespan continues to be extended. And, since the majority of the major consequences occur in women over 65 years old, these women are eligible for Medicare, which is funded mostly by taxes passed on to the American public.

This phenomenon is why I consider the osteoporosis epidemic to be the greatest hidden tax burden on working Americans. Unless something is done, and soon, the crisis will only worsen, and ever larger numbers of women will be killed and disfigured by osteoporosis.

Who is to blame? There have been no major congressional meetings, resolutions or laws to which the evolution of this hidden tax may be attributed. Does the blame fall on the medical establishment? Mostly. Does it also fall on the health insurance carriers? Certainly. Does it fall on the elderly? Partly. Does it fall on the government? Yes, as a result of the traditionally meager funding of medical research on women's health issues. In recent years, however, with the increasing focus on health, fitness and women's health issues in particular, there have no longer been any valid excuses for women and their physicians to ignore this silent killer known as osteoporosis.

One way to think about osteoporosis is to consider an analogy of a house's wooden frame structure. Osteoporosis may be likened to the effect that termites, left untreated, have on the house's structure. Eventually, the roof begins to cave in due to the weakening of support. Unfortunately, by the time one actually sees a swarm of termites in or

Introduction

around a house, substantial damage has probably already occurred. Before one even buys a house, a termite inspection is required as a preventive measure. That's because we are all well aware of the damage that the termite process can cause.

Isn't it a shame that we inspect and take care of the wooden structure of our houses more than we do our own bones? No matter how much money one spends on the external beauty of a house infected with termites, left undiagnosed and untreated, the house will eventually collapse.

Many women over 45 years old have no trouble spending substantial amounts of money on their external beauty — hair and nail appointments, makeup and beauty aids, breast implants, liposuction, facelifts and other cosmetic surgery — yet their bone structures may be crumbling away. Why not keep up the condition of our internal bone structure as well as our external appearance?

Over the past few decades, American women have attained a greater average adult height than ever before, but the average coffin size for women is perhaps shorter than it was over a century ago. This seeming paradox can be explained by the osteoporosis epidemic, plain and simple. In other words, American women are growing taller during their adolescence and early adult years, but ultimately they are shrinking more in the postmenopausal years, making them shorter at death.

Must the medical establishment, which did not even consider postmenopausal osteoporosis a disease until recently, wait until we are burying elderly white women in small boxes before it learns what was taught over fifty years ago by published medical pioneers?

Even our concepts about aging women have been influenced by osteoporosis. Who ever referred to an elderly woman as a "big old lady"? Obviously, she tends to wear the label of "little old lady." If she is little it may well be because the osteoporosis process made her that way. And most white women, if they live long enough, will come to wear this label unless the medical establishment reverses the current mainstream concepts and therapies for osteoporosis.

How can it be that postmenopausal osteoporosis is more common

Introduction

in white women than many of the more highly publicized diseases such as breast cancer and AIDS combined?

Within this book the facts of how the osteoporosis epidemic occurred are presented in a truthful manner — which may make many physicians, politicians, and national women's groups uneasy. A retrospective look at the historical facts, especially those which were rebuffed or ignored, is often a hard pill to swallow.

Within this text, the evolution of the osteoporosis epidemic is examined in terms of the early historical factors, the period of sex steroid experimentation on women, the influences of false medical dogma, the current attitudes of a variety of physicians and the attempts to correct the mistakes of past and present via reeducation. Then, and only then, can the reader become educated to exactly where the responsibility for this epidemic lies today on the public, political, medical and legal playing fields.

Other topics will include the relationship between the sex steroids and basic bone metabolism, the correct methods for the diagnosis and treatments of osteoporosis, questions and answers regarding specific osteoporosis cases and interviews with a number of physicians regarding the disease.

I believe that this medical epidemic was made by humans, who entered the early stages of the epidemic with certain prejudices, propensities and predispositions. From this early platform, "medical authorities" constructed a picture of the practice of medicine the way that they wanted it practiced. This epidemic is the sum of facts noted, facts ignored and the subsequent false medical dogma which grew out of such a platform. And, underlying this medical epidemic is a characteristic common to most epidemics: its predictability in retrospect.

Medical mistakes often occur when facts are ignored or slanted. Then, the medical textbooks can become laden with incorrect statements which are taught to medical students, medical residents and practicing physicians without any direct reference or footnote. And once these major medical textbooks promote these mistakes, subsequent editions of the same books simply tend to promulgate much of it over and over again without question.

Introduction

It is my intent that the pages which follow, condensed from interdisciplinary study, personal medical experience, personal dedication and personal medical publications, will contribute something of value toward a solution to the osteoporosis epidemic. I believe, more strongly than I have believed anything else in my medical journey, that I know a solution. This solution is derived from the long-ignored scientific publications, of the pioneers in much earlier medical times.

These pages will show that even the FDA perhaps knew and approved of the solution up until 1981, and then effectively tossed it away. In the case of osteoporosis, medical mistakes became the major cause, osteoporosis was the resulting epidemic, and culturing human genius will be the solution.

Culturing human genius through profound study is what Alexander Hamilton (1757–1804) had in mind when he wrote, "Men give me credit for genius; but all the genius I have lies in this: When I have a subject on hand, I study it profoundly." That is what we must do with the subject of osteoporosis.

Chapter 1

Building Blocks of the Epidemic

To identify the building blocks from which the current osteoporosis epidemic is constructed it is necessary to take a trip back in time and to examine the medical mistakes and medical policies which led to perhaps the largest human health epidemic the United States has ever seen. The trip back is not difficult to perform, but it does require an examination of the old medical books and medical journals.

To completely understand the mistakes which were made, one may in addition have to enter the role of a philosopher. It can be difficult to distinguish among opinions, emotions and philosophies based on differences that may be subtle. With any controversial issue, these basic differences, however difficult to discern, provide the basis for solutions. The usual opinions may lack the facts, and emotions tend to override the more factual opinions. However, a philosophical approach is attained only after the passage of time has allowed the philosopher to study and reflect on an issue from many perspectives.

As H.G. Wells wrote in *The Mind at the End of Its Tether* (1946):

Osteoporosis

The philosophical mind is not what people would call a healthy buoyant mind. That "healthy mind" takes life as it finds it and troubles no more about that. None of us start life as philosophers. We become philosophers sooner or later, or we die before we become philosophical. The realization of limitation and frustration is the beginning of the bitter wisdom of philosophy, and of this, that "healthy mind" by its innate gift for incoherence and piecemeal evasion and credulity, never knows. Mind may be at the end of its tether and it is that every day drama that will be the normal makeup of life and there is nothing else to replace it.

The everyday drama of the osteoporosis epidemic may have an easy and inexpensive solution, but for now it is ubiquitous and day by day it drains the money and life of American white women and the public in general.

It takes nothing more than an experienced eye to spot this disease process in elderly women. The loss of adult height, the condensing of a woman's trunk making her appear as if she is all legs, the characteristic slumping of the shoulders, the humplike appearance of her upper back and neck, and the hemlines of her skirt or dress which hangs longer in the front than in the back are seen in every grocery store every day in America.

The medical establishment has, however, failed to combat this disease. Common sense tells us that the medical establishment has been misguided regarding the proper diagnosis, treatment and reversal of the osteoporosis condition. The millions of women who are living with osteoporosis and the millions who have died from its consequences represent a major embarrassment to an increasing number of practicing physicians.

With most diseases, physicians often think to themselves, What made this patient wait so long before seeking medical attention? But with osteoporosis, the patients have been there all along and in their offices for other medical conditions. The patients have developed osteoporosis right under the physicians' noses, and most have developed the attitude that there is nothing that can be done about it anyway.

Building Blocks of the Epidemic

Even postmenopausal women physicians who have signs of osteoporosis themselves tend to believe that they cannot help themselves, much less their postmenopausal women patients.

Some of the false ideas which were taught in medical schools during the 1970s and beyond and which served as the basic building blocks for the modern osteoporosis epidemic are listed below. In the chapters which follow, direct quotations from major medical textbooks and medical journals of earlier times will provide examples of how these notions have been promoted.

Among these myths are the following:

• Calcium supplements should not be prescribed to women patients because additional calcium in the diet may cause kidney stones.

• Estrogens should not be prescribed to postmenopausal women because the adverse effects are greater than the beneficial effects.

• Testosterone and anabolic-androgenic steroids (androgens) are male sex steroid hormones with little, if any, psychological or physiological importance to women.

• Osteoporosis is a normal aging process in women, not a disease condition.

These truisms were taught to decades of medical students and medical doctors, and much of the medical establishment has been misled by them for a significant period of time. Even with the recent efforts to reeducate physicians, many of them still hold on to their old and outdated practices.

For example, when I recently lectured to physicians in my local area on the treatment of osteoporosis, I was met with a mixed response: some thought this new approach to treating and reversing osteoporosis was one of the best lectures they had heard, while others considered my research too controversial and my presentation too outspoken. The latter group, if they insist on following only conventional wisdom, will keep on missing the diagnosis and ineffectively treating osteoporosis in their women patients. This is a sad and, in my opinion, unconscionable fact.

Today, medical, surgical, dental, osteopathic, chiropractic, and psychiatric physicians are making fortunes attending to the fractures, pain and mental disturbances associated with postmenopausal osteoporosis.

Psychologists and psychiatrists are making a living dealing with women who suffer mental conditions directly related to a diminishment or complete lack of sex steroid production, but most do not even consider this phenomenon and its subsequent effects on personality, sense of well-being and behavior.

Dental physicians observe on X-rays the deterioration of the jaw bones of many of their elderly white patients, but very few ever refer the patient for an osteoporosis evaluation.

Chiropractic physicians see osteoporosis on spine X-rays and then go ahead and manipulate the spine anyway, sometimes causing microfractures in the bones of the spine in some cases.

Over the years, osteoporosis became something of a pervasive secret amongst medically trained professionals, and there was really no segment of the medical establishment to which one could point as an osteoporosis expert or board certified in osteoporosis.

The result of this predicament was that osteoporosis became a "Humpty Dumpty" condition for many older women: all the king's horses and all the king's assorted specialists could not put them back together again. Many of today's physicians are typically ignoring the dramatic loss of adult height and loss of bone mineral density in their postmenopausal patients. In fact, many medical charts are completely void of a very cost-effective measurement: accurately measuring adult height. Many physicians devote little attention to osteoporosis because they believe there is no treatment which can reverse it.

The osteoporosis epidemic is surely serious enough to qualify for a major focus of public attention, but it has never been treated as a political issue and has never received heavy media coverage. Menopausal issues tend to be silent killers which attack women later in life in a variety of ways. In simple numbers of victims, the chronic pain and eventual premature deaths caused by osteoporo overshadow the effects of all cancers in women.

Is it that osteoporosis is not "glitzy" enough to receive the media attention which other more controversial or more politically polarized diseases receive, even though it affects more than 25 million Americans? Gail Sheehy, author of a 1994 book entitled *Menopause*, states that the condition of osteoporosis "has not been worthy of recognition" and "represents another political medical scandal regarding women's health issues."

I concur. What are the facts behind this political medical scandal? Read on.

Chapter 2

The Period of Sex Steroid Experimentation

Introduction

In this chapter the history of sex steroid experimentation on women will be examined in detail. As this chapter will show, as soon as the experimentation began, so did the medical political platforms begin to form. After all, it has been difficult for the medical profession to reach real comprehension of how the sex steroids work physiologically in both women and men.

And perhaps nothing in human physiology and psychology has ever been so intriguing, yet misunderstood, as the role of the sex steroids in the human body. The early medical experimentation with these steroids engendered all sorts of dogma which came to be more influential than actual medical science in the development of the osteoporosis epidemic. How can it be that sex steroids are important in this way?

Sex steroid production by a woman's ovaries is intertwined with normal bone metabolism, bone density, and bone strength. Once the production of these sex steroids diminishes, so usually does the strength, density and integrity of her bones begin to decline. In many women, the years leading up to menopause (perimenopausal years) and the postmenopausal years are part of a continuum of diminished sex steroid production. This is a natural process which has significant consequences both physically and mentally. Men go through a sort of menopause of their own, but the reduction in the sex steroids usually occurs over a much longer period of time.

About a decade or so before the actual menopause proper, a woman's ovaries may begin to produce less and less of the sex steroids. Previously normal menstrual cycles may become irregular as the ovarian function begins to "sputter." The ovaries usually make three classes of sex steroid hormones: estrogenic steroids (estrogens), progesterogenic steroids (progesterones), and anabolic-androgenic steroids (androgens). The perimenopausal sputtering may cause a diminished production of all three classes of these sex steroids. Which class of sex steroids diminishes earliest is still a mystery, and it may be that the androgens actually are the ones that diminish before the others. This has caused some authors recently to refer to the perimenopausal years as "andropause."

After a year or so without menstrual cycles, a woman officially may be labeled as postmenopausal. By then, the production of all three classes of the sex steroids has greatly diminished, and they will remain diminished for the remainder of her life unless they are therapeutically replaced. These sex steroids are important for both the physical and mental well-being of a woman, and many physical and mental ailments are associated with this diminished sex hormone production during the perimenopausal and postmenopausal years.

Many women can expect to live over half of their adult lives suffering from the sequelae of ovarian involution. So to treat many of the physical and mental ailments associated with a diminished sex steroid production, it makes sense that therapy utilizing the proper sex steroid replacement would be beneficial. In fact, in the May 1995 issue of *Prevention* magazine, Dr. Gambrell of the Medical College of Georgia, who trained with Dr. Robert Greenblatt (see Acknowledgments),

The Period of Sex Steroid Experimentation

supports this concept entirely. He, like the present author, tailors the sex steroid replacement in his women patients by utilizing all three of the classes of the sex steroids which the ovaries used to make.

Perhaps the most important of these classes of sex steroids for bone integrity are the androgens and estrogens. Androgens directly stimulate the bone forming cells (osteoblasts). Estrogens inhibit the bone dissolving cells (osteoclasts). The basics of the roles of the sex steroids will be discussed in greater detail in this book, but it is important to introduce this concept now so that the reader can fully appreciate the importance of the remainder of this chapter.

In this chapter, as with the following chapters, certain dogmatic medical statements will be quoted from the most authoritative authors of medical textbooks and medical publications of decades ago. This author, along with his peers, was taught the misinformation contained in several of these quotes. Later these quotations will be used as a basis for discussion regarding the historical factors which caused the osteoporosis epidemic. In some cases, the reader may find it hard to believe that these statements were actually made in medical texts, but I hope the reader takes these quotes on face value, because they indeed exist and were taught as facts. But first, let us set the stage for the period of sex steroid experimentation by looking briefly at the medical front prior to the discovery of the sex steroids.

Beginning of a Misunderstanding

Many people believe that our present medical establishment has existed for a longer period of time than it actually has. When sex steroid experimentation on women began in the late 1930s, the medical practice was only in its infancy.

At the beginning of the twentieth century the average lifespan for a woman was about 50 years, which was also the average age of menopause. Therefore, at that time there was very little known about postmenopausal health conditions. There was no such thing as health insurance, Medicare, worker's compensation, prescription medicines or medical bureaucracy. Almost all physicians were men.

A significant percentage of Americans were drug addicts even before the pharmaceutical industry had manufactured the first drug from chemical reactions. For instance, one in every 400 Americans was addicted to some form of opium at that time — a greater percentage than at any other time in American history. Also, the percentage of Americans who smoked marijuana at the turn of the century rivaled that of the 1960s, which is popularly identified as the period of greatest usage. Yet no drug had been synthesized by chemical reactions, and medical physicians of the times had very few drugs or "elixirs" available to them for the treatment of medical conditions. What was available had been obtained from extracts of plants, herbs and fungi, such as poppy (opium), corn (ethanol), cactus (peyote), mushrooms (hallucinogens), marijuana and tobacco.

Shortly before and during World War II, biology and biochemistry began to change the face of the medical practice forever. Actually, the biochemical aspects of science were far ahead of the medical profession in general. A variety of drugs were synthesized by biochemists in the expanding pharmaceutical industry. All sorts of diseases were being described by the medical profession, based mostly on observation and physical examination.

Patients were in need of medical help, and as the drugs became available, physicians were placed in a mode of clinical experimentation with few or no laboratory tests available to back them up. And at that time, there were only a few federal regulations regarding prescription drugs, and there was no FDA or Drug Enforcement Agency.

With the field of biology advancing rapidly, a profusion of drugs were chemically synthesized and brought onto the medical scene very quickly. Drug manufacturing severely outpaced the other areas of medical technology so that many drugs were used on people before their effects were fully known; the result was a period of clinical experimentation. So-called medical authorities began, often arbitrarily, to place all of these new drugs into various classes and to give these

The Period of Sex Steroid Experimentation

classes names based on what they knew about the drugs' effects at that time.

There were mistakes made, and errors in nomenclature were plentiful during this period. For example, testosterone was called "the male sex steroid hormone." Most physicians even today refer to testosterone and other androgens in this misleading manner, even though it is now known that testosterone and other androgens flow in the bloodstreams of every normal man and woman.

Likewise, estrogenic steroids were called "the female sex steroid hormones" and are still known as such by most physicians today even though they too are present in people of both sexes.

With regard to the sex steroids, the human body is very parsimonious, for it utilizes the same sex steroids in both men and women. But, it was these early historical mistakes in the nomenclature of the sex steroids that began a misunderstanding that would allow the osteoporosis epidemic to grow unchecked decades later.

In other words, medical science ignited the flame early on by incorrectly naming the sex steroids. The early researchers wanted medical science to permit the sex steroids to be named in such a manner that men had one type of sex steroid while women had another. But no matter how much they wanted it that way, it just was not so.

Early Clinical Experimentation with Androgens

The first sex steroid hormone synthesized by chemical reactions was testosterone in 1935. Both a German research group and a Swiss research group received the Nobel Prize by synthesizing testosterone from cholesterol, although the German researchers declined their award for political reasons.

Physicians were eager to treat a variety of medical diseases and conditions with testosterone in the 1940s, and later with its chemical cousins, synthetic anabolic-androgenic steroids, in the 1950s and 1960s. One of the diseases which responded to treatment with androgens was osteoporosis. The present author has written two textbooks about the various diseases which androgen therapy was beneficial in treating in both genders: *Anabolic Steroids and the Athlete* (1982) and *Macho Medicine: A History of the Anabolic Steroid Epidemic* (1991). The other sex steroids, which play an important role with women's health conditions, including osteoporosis, were synthesized years later.

Medical science today should be fully informed that the functioning human ovaries produce three major classes of sex steroids. But surprisingly, some physicians tend to forget or overlook this fact, even today. Most know very little about androgens and their effects on women.

By retracing the historical footsteps with regard to the synthesis of and early clinical experimentation with the sex steroids, the reader can gain a better understanding of the controversies which currently surround the use of sex steroid replacement for the treatment of osteoporosis.

The importance of synthetic testosterone and other androgens for osteoporosis therapy in both women and men was appreciated by the medical profession in the early 1940s, but harnessing these powerful sex steroids for appropriate medical use presented problems.

Just by "shooting from the hip," not knowing the proper dose or treatment regimens, and having no way to measure the appropriate blood testing, clinical physicians of this period indicated that the key to treating osteoporosis was linked to testosterone and other androgen therapy.

Testosterone and other androgens possess a major characteristic which threw their use into conflict with the mores of the times: these sex steroids are the natural chemical aphrodisiacs in both men and women, as was scientifically and irrefutably proven by distinguished medical researchers in the early 1940s. In the first medical book written about its use, published in 1945, testosterone was labeled "medical dynamite" and "sexual TNT" by some prominent physicians at that time.

Since there were as yet no laboratory tests available to determine the appropriate dosage of testosterone to administer to a patient, treatment with testosterone was largely a matter of guesswork. Some physicians of that period tended to give too much testosterone, and adverse effects arose. Sometimes the dose given was several times too much.

By the early 1940s physicians began to become polarized in their views of testosterone and other androgen therapies in women, as became evident from a crossfire of different viewpoints expressed in articles and letters published in the medical journals. For instance, a letter from Robert B. Greenblatt, M.D., in a 1942 issue of the *Journal of Clinical Endocrinology* read in part,

> In a recent letter to the Editor which sharply condemns the use of androgens in the practice of gynecology ... one point which is fundamental and with which none will take issue is that the excessive use of any pharmacologic agent, hormonal or otherwise, is harmful. The voices that have been raised against the use of androgens in the female arise from the concept that gonadal hormones should be sex specific. ... Pharmacologically effective doses of testosterone propionate, which are far below the virilizing level, have been employed in several hundred cases by our group.

Dr. Greenblatt knew that there was no such thing as the gender specific nature of the sex hormones, but this quotation from him clearly showed that some physicians were already committed to the idea that so-called male sex steroids should be used only in men and the so-called female sex steroids only in females. Dr. Greenblatt knew that all classes of sex steroids were common in both men and women. Other physicians echoed Dr. Greenblatt's work and policies:

> One should be careful in condemning the general use of a valuable drug, like testosterone, just because some practitioners abuse it. ... Should condemn the improper use of any new drug by such practitioners, but not the drug itself [Alex Goldman, M.D., *J. Clinical Endocrinology* (1942)].

> The use of androgenic hormones for the relief of varied functional gynecologic disorders, including the menopause, has now been thoroughly accepted [Melvyn Berlind, M.D., *J. Clinical Endocrinology* (1941)].

Early battle lines were drawn over the use of testosterone and other androgens as therapy for women. But it was much too early to be drawing such battle lines, for the research was only in its early phase.

The conflict quickly became political and dogmatic in nature. Apparently, some physicians were abusing androgen therapy in some of their patients by utilizing much higher doses than others had found to be appropriate. There was some guesswork involved, for strict guidelines had not been developed yet. In women patients, deepening of the voice, acne and some facial hair were common complaints when the higher doses were administered.

Testosterone and androgen therapy, like any other hormonal therapy, can have adverse effects if they are prescribed in too large a dose. By way of comparison, imagine doubling a diabetic's dose of the hormone insulin for a week or two. The results could be lethal.

Perhaps the major point of political, social and moral contention dealt with the effect of androgens on sexual drive and sexual pleasure, especially when the doses were too large. Physicians of this period began to feel more and more uneasy about administering any drug that increased the sex drive and orgasmic response, especially in women. At the time, the female orgasmic response was poorly understood and was essentially a taboo subject both medically and socially speaking.

By holding on to the concept that sex steroids should be gender specific, some physicians *wanted* the so-called female sex steroids (estrogens) to control the sex drive and sexual responses in women, despite the definitive research that indicated otherwise.

By the late 1940s testosterone and other androgen therapies were largely abandoned by the medical community, even though they were known to play an important role in bone metabolism and in the treatment of osteoporosis. Factors contributing to this "black-balling" included the following:

• The early nomenclature mistakes made some physicians ignore the published research and hold to their desires to make sex steroid therapy gender specific.

• Some of the early physicians used excessive doses in their androgen treatment regimens in women. There were no laboratory values to assist them and there were no strict guidelines for androgen therapy at that time. Some physicians feared that they would make men out of their women patients.

• The libido-enhancing effects which androgen therapy could cause prompted some physicians to worry about its effects on women and society; they thought that it may have bawdy overtones. Some may have felt that this sort of effect precluded androgen therapy in treatment of diseases and conditions with which it had been shown to be beneficial.

Authors of medical textbooks, influenced by the above concerns, attempted to wipe the clinical use of testosterone and other anabolic-androgenic steroids off the scientific map permanently. But a few prominent physicians continued to believe in their work. Even Sigmund Freud had become "firmly convinced that one day mental disturbances would be treated with hormones or similar substances."

Without a doubt, sex steroid therapy was the most volatile topic in medicine for decades. The effects of the poorly grounded fears about its use could still be seen in the medical textbooks decades later, as illustrated by the following quotation from *Harrison's Principles of Internal Medicine*, Eighth Edition (1977), the "bible" of internal medicine:

> Estrogens act by decreasing the rate of bone resorption, but bone formation does not increase, and usually decreases. Thus, estrogens produce significant, although modest, calcium

retention, decrease the difference between formation and resorption, and therefore tend to retard the progress of osteoporosis, but they are not capable of restoring skeletal mass. ... With testosterone preparations and anabolic steroids there is no advantage to their use in women in view of their masculinizing properties. There is also no proved advantage to combinations of estrogens and androgens.

The book containing this passage has taught the majority of the nation's medical students, medical interns, medical residents and physicians. There are no footnotes or references directly relating to the quote; the information was simply presented as fact.

The sentences on estrogens and their effect on bone metabolism are correct according to the scientific knowledge available then and today. A discussion of the historical factors regarding the use of estrogens will be presented later in this chapter.

The sentences regarding testosterone and anabolic steroids are incorrect, however and were presented without acknowledging the proven scientific research which indicated contrary results. Thanks to such incomplete or inaccurate information, the use of these important sex steroids in women patients came to be frowned upon and the osteoporosis epidemic was the result.

Regardless of what the medical establishment was trying to do with androgen therapy, for society, nature would take its usual pathway. Once the word about sex steroids was publicly known, a variety of hucksters began selling supplements which were claimed to contain sex steroids, including testosterone. This phenomenon became so widespread that the FDA, still in its infancy, placed a nationwide ban on the manufacturing and selling of these steroid supplements in the mid–1940s.

But the clinical and scientific work continued. Published findings of the early clinical experimentation indicated that testosterone and other androgens were used successfully in a variety of disease states and other medical conditions, having positive effects for the following:

The Period of Sex Steroid Experimentation

- underweight patients;
- patients with rheumatoid arthritis;
- surgical patients during recovery;
- patients with myelofibrosis;
- patients with various anemias;
- patients with osteoporosis;
- male patients with male menopause;
- female patients with gynecologic disturbances, including menopausal symptoms, endometriosis and lack of libido;
- male and female patients with angina pectoris (chest pain);
- male and female patients with hypertension;
- male and female patients with hyperlipidemia;
- children as a growth stimulator;
- patients with Raynaud's syndrome;
- enhancement of muscle mass, strength and athletic performance;
- premature babies, both male and female, to stimulate growth and development and reduce the stay in the hospital;
- male boys to treat enuresis (bed wetting);
- a variety of mental states, including depression and actual psychotic illnesses;
- male patients with impotence;
- boys with delayed puberty;
- suntanning enhancement in women; and
- patients with depressed immune systems.

The clinical studies conducted during this period indicated that testosterone and other androgens had some powerful effects on the human body, but it proved difficult to convert those effects into accepted methods for treating disease conditions once medical politics had caused these therapies to fall out of favor. Perhaps, if some of the current medical technology could be applied to androgen therapy today, more specific indications could be found for these steroids in modern medicine.

American physicians and scientists were not the only ones conducting early clinical experimentation on testosterone and other androgens. Several reports surfaced which claimed that German soldiers, especially the Gestapo, were taking these steroids during World War II. American propaganda depicted these Germans as strong, overly aggressive and highly sexually driven. Jewish people in German concentration camps were said to have served as subjects for Nazi experiments with these sex steroids. Even Adolf Hitler was injected with these sex steroids, according to the records of his personal physician which were finally released in the late 1980s and published by the American Medical Association.

Perhaps the greatest reason that clinical research and experimentation with testosterone and other androgens began to slow to a trickle was the bad reputation these steroids were gaining as a result of the athletic use and abuse of them in the Olympic Games during the 1950s. Worldwide research was conducted to determine the effects that these sex steroids had on athletic performance. After 20 or so studies were published on the effects which these sex steroids had on athletic performance, the international medical and sports medicine organizations proclaimed that these steroids were nothing more than mere placebos for athletes. This assertion proved to be incorrect, but it had its influence anyway. As Geoffrey Redmond, M.D., writes in *The Good News About Women's Hormones*, "We all believed that testosterone levels were maximal, and giving more would not make any difference. This belief was incorrect."

Considering all of these problems and abuses, it is no wonder that synthetic testosterone and other androgens got off to a less than auspicious start. But recall that it was never the steroids which were bad or evil; androgens exist in everyone's body. Testosterone was perhaps the first hormone ever discovered and synthesized from chemical reactions, and the result was a progression of inappropriate medical, political and social reactions, due mostly to the timing of the discovery and the shortcomings of medical technology at that time.

The Period of Sex Steroid Experimentation

Many factors collided and resulted in tainting the research findings of the early clinical experimentation so that medical politics could discourage further clinical use and research. Outright lies about these sex steroids became commonplace.

By 1963, the pharmaceutical industry had synthesized nearly 20 different synthetic forms of testosterone and anabolic-androgenic steroids for clinical use in the United States and abroad, and the FDA-approved promotional literature and package inserts regarding these sex steroids clearly indicated that these steroids were indicated for treating osteoporosis in women and men. Yet the accurate and definitive bone mineral density testing machines used currently to detect osteoporosis had not been invented. Androgens were used to treat osteoporosis for decades.

As late as 1981, Winthrop Pharmaceutical Company promoted an anabolic-androgenic steroid, Winstrol (stanozolol) to the nation's physicians for the treatment of postmenopausal osteoporosis. This author was a resident at the time, and can remember when the Winthrop representatives sent samples of Winstrol to American physicians and made sales calls to promote its use for the treatment of osteoporosis. Package inserts for the drug indicated this use as well quoting the FDA's classification of Winstrol as "probably" effective as adjunctive therapy in treating osteoporosis.

The last effort to promote anabolic-androgenic steroids for the treatment of osteoporosis essentially fell on deaf ears, largely because the patents had expired on all of the testosterone and anabolic-androgenic steroid preparations which were available in the 1960s. There was no more incentive for the pharmaceutical companies to continue to promote these products to physicians since they could now be manufactured by any other pharmaceutical company.

Then in the early 1980s, Congress passed legislation which allowed for makers of generic pharmaceuticals to copy the patents of the major pharmaceutical companies and mass produce these products.

As the patents expired for sex steroids like Winstrol, the indication of their use to treat osteoporosis was dropped. Orthopedic

Osteoporosis

surgeons continued to make a fortune performing surgery on the elderly men and women who sustained osteoporosis-related hip fractures.

One may ask, why would the nation's orthopedic surgeons even want to prescribe a sex steroid to treat osteoporosis when they could make so much money from the surgical measures associated with osteoporosis? Besides, their textbooks in medical school had taught them that osteoporosis could not be reversed and that androgen therapy was certainly not even worth considering. Therefore, the last-ditch efforts of the pharmaceutical companies to educate the physicians who practiced in the early 1980s failed.

In the early 1980s, the FDA was performing a task which had been assigned to it: to "clean up" the approved indications for many drugs. In doing so the FDA dropped the indication for anabolic-androgenic steroids, so today the *Physician's Desk Reference* contains absolutely no mention of the use of this class of sex steroids for osteoporosis therapy. The FDA dropped this previously approved indication nearly a decade prior to the development of the definitive osteoporosis scanning machines which are now proving that androgens can reverse major losses in bone mineral density in patients with osteoporosis.

This author watched all of this happen. It was demoralizing to the point of making me much less proud to be a physician when I watched the FDA toss away this information and knowledge. And to think, I once served as an expert witness for the FDA in federal court on the very topic of anabolic-androgenic steroids!

For a moment, let us pretend that anabolic-androgenic steroids were recently discovered and the current medical technology was available today to give this class of drugs a fair test, for once. Let's pretend that Winstrol was the best candidate for the reversal and potential cure of osteoporosis and that it was a brand new drug. What would happen? Let's suppose that we chose one of Winstrol's functions and named it an "osteoblast stimulator" instead of an anabolic-androgenic steroid; then we would not have to deal with the troubled history of this class of sex steroids, but could just focus on its

The Period of Sex Steroid Experimentation

effects in treating osteoporosis. The following events would probably occur:

• Winstrol would become one of the most heavily prescribed drugs in the United States;
• Winstrol therapy, in combination with an estrogen, would ultimately save billions of dollars annually in health care expenditures;
• Winstrol therapy, in combination with an estrogen, would have a major impact on reducing the pain, suffering and surgical procedures in American white women; and,
• Winstrol therapy, in combination with an estrogen, would help prolong the quality and quantity of life for millions of American women.

Basic Physiology of Androgens

It has been known for decades that several bodily functions are controlled either directly or indirectly by testosterone and anabolic-androgenic steroids within the human body. Some of these bodily functions have been artificially delineated as either anabolic (to build) or androgenic (man-like) characteristics. The various anabolic-androgenic steroids differ in their abilities to produce the anabolic functions over the androgenic functions. Some of these anabolic and androgenic functions are listed below.

Anabolic Functions

• Increased skeletal muscle mass and strength in both males and females, especially combined with regular strength training
• Increased hemoglobin concentration in males which helps with maximum aerobic capacity and endurance
• Decreased body fat percentage
• Increased calcium deposition in the bones through osteoblast

Table 1. Therapeutic Index for Some Anabolic-Androgenic Steroids*

Trade Name	Generic Name	Original Manufacturer	Therapeutic Index
Depo-Testosterone	testosterone	Upjohn	1
Halotestin	fluoroxymesterone	Upjohn	2–6
Dianabol	methandrostenolone	Ciba	2–7
Anadrol	oxymesterone	Searle	3–8
Deca-Durabolin	nandrolone decanoate	Organon	11–12
Winstrol	stanolozol	Winthrop	15–20

*taken from Taylor, W. N., *Anabolic Steroids and the Athlete* (1982).

stimulation which leads to increased bone mineral density in both males and females

• Increased total body nitrogen retention

• Increased retention of several electrolytes

Androgenic Functions

• Increased density of body and facial hair

• Development and pattern of pubic hair

• Deepened tone of the voice

• Increased oil production of the sebaceous glands

• Increased libido and awakening of sexual interest in both males and females

The complete separation of these two basic types of anabolic and androgenic functions in the human has never been fully accomplished by any natural or synthetic testosterone or anabolic-androgenic steroids, but certain products do lean much more strongly toward anabolic functions. A ratio of the anabolic to androgenic functions has been termed the *therapeutic index* for that particular sex steroid by a variety of scientific techniques. The therapeutic indexes for testosterone and some other anabolic-androgenic steroids are shown for comparison in Table 1.

The therapeutic index is useful in selecting an anabolic-androgenic steroid with the greatest margin of safety. For instance, in treating osteoporosis in women, choosing an anabolic-androgenic steroid with a high therapeutic index, given in the lowest possible dose for osteoblast stimulation, can help ensure that the desired effect does not come at the expense of unwanted side effects.

Some of the results of scientific studies using small doses of anabolic-androgenic steroid replacement in women will be discussed later in Chapter 4.

Early Clinical Experimentation with Estrogenic Steroids

As previously mentioned, the functioning human ovaries make three classes of sex steroid hormones. The two classes which are the most important for maintaining bone mineral density and bone strength are the anabolic-androgenic steroids and the estrogenic steroids. The former stimulate the osteoblast and the latter inhibit the osteoclast.

The history of medical use of the estrogenic steroids, like that of testosterone and the other anabolic-androgenic steroids, has been troubled.

Nonetheless, as the decades went by since estrogens were first used clinically, and most postmenopausal women went untreated with estrogens, clinicians began to realize that the postmenopausal women treated with estrogens experienced fewer mental and physical ailments than those who were treated.

However, the prevailing medical dogma which came out of the early period of experimentation with estrogens is exemplified by the following textbook quotation:

> Mild depression is not uncommon in menopausal women, its frequency tending to be inversely proportional to the patient's understanding of menopausal physiology. A "menopause

syndrome" in a psychiatric sense appears to be nonexistent. Women with anxiety neurosis, hysteria, phobic states, hypochondriasis, or obsessive-compulsive neurological illness during the menopause are generally found to have had the illness earlier in life. Psychological problems related to the menopause per se are common in the 40–55 year old group and relate to the "empty nest" syndrome; responsibility for the care of adolescent children and aging parents; ungratified sexuality; fears of obesity, cancer, and loss of sexual attractiveness; and the fear of having to ultimately depend on children or charity.

This list, from *Harrison's Principles of Internal Medicine*, eighth edition (1977), does not speak very well to middle-aged women, does it? And it ignores the fact that some middle-aged men have all of the same feelings at times. Actually, Dr. Harrison used the above paragraph to summarize some of the mental and physical conditions associated with the perimenopausal and postmenopausal states, but he came to incorrect assessments.

This description tends to designate perimenopausal and postmenopausal women as "psych cases." Moreover, it ignores the facts (known in 1977) that the mental and physical menopausal symptoms can be related to a great degree to a diminished sex steroid production.

During medical school, I saw hundreds of middle-aged women with mental and physical complaints during their perimenopausal and postmenopausal years referred inappropriately to psychiatrists. How did the treatment and misunderstanding of the menopausal states get to this point by the late 1970s?

Perhaps the first estrogenic steroid that became available for treating postmenopausal women with osteoporosis was Premarin, a product derived from the urine of pregnant horses. Officially, Premarin is considered "equine urine-derived conjugated estrogens." It is still manufactured today, decades later, by the same basic methods that were used originally. It contains a mixture of dozens of sex steroid molecules which a woman's body may have no use for, including a few

The Period of Sex Steroid Experimentation

that are made only by horses for horses. Humans do not make them at all.

Some of these sex steroids may produce adverse effects in some women — sometimes in normally prescribed doses, but especially in higher doses. The term "conjugated" in the clinical designation means that the horse's liver chemically adds certain molecules, known as side chains, to make the estrogenic steroids more soluble in urine, so that the horse can excrete them in the urine as byproducts. These sex steroid byproducts constitute the chemical basis of Premarin.

The use of Premarin in women during the early scientific studies may have tainted the findings and conclusions regarding the use of estrogenic steroid replacement for decades. Some of the claimed adverse effects, such as breast cancer or uterine cancer, may have been caused in some women by a mixture of horse urine byproducts, and not by the true human estrogens at all. Questions about the early experimentation with horse urine byproducts may never be completely cleared up by future research.

But in all fairness, Premarin was available for clinical use, still is, and has had its place in medical history. In my opinion Premarin has been clinically obsolete for several years, but prescription writing is often a habitual thing for physicians, and the fact is that Premarin is still the most prescribed estrogenic steroid replacement therapy for American women today.

There were other factors which tainted the early clinical experimentation with estrogenic steroids. For instance, the practicing physicians prescribed estrogenic steroids in excessive doses, and adverse effects were definitely seen. Many physicians then began to back away from estrogen replacement therapy, and this movement was supported by the major medical textbooks.

By the 1970s medical opinion was definitely turning against the use of estrogen replacement therapy. Some of the reasons were as follows:

• The most common estrogens which were prescribed were horse urine byproducts containing over 50 types of estrogenic steroids instead of a single synthetic copy of the most important human estrogen.

• The prescribed doses of these horse urine byproducts were often too large, and adverse effects arose.

• The medical confusion which surrounded the concepts of the perimenopausal and postmenopausal states made all physicians begin to look incompetent.

This movement away from estrogen replacement not only fueled the current osteoporosis epidemic, but perhaps discouraged the pharmaceutical industry from developing synthetic versions of the human estrogens.

Previous scientific publications had showed that many of the menopausal symptoms relate directly to a sex steroid deficiency, but with the movement away from prescribing estrogen replacement, the authors of medical textbooks had to come up with some explanation as to why menopausal women were having problems. The most revered medical textbook of the 1970s suggested that cultural and environmental factors were partially to blame. I object to blaming hot flashes, postmenopausal depression and osteoporosis on cultural and environmental causes when ovarian cessation and sex steroid deficiency are known facts of menopause.

Most of the longitudinal studies which showed that estrogen-taking women could suffer adverse effects were performed with horse urine byproducts. What if these studies had been done with correct dosage of synthetic copies of the natural estrogens in humans? Would the clinical experimentation period have taken a different course? I believe it would have.

Thanks to modern technology, the actual natural estrogenic steroid that the human ovaries produce in the greatest quantities has been synthesized and prepared for oral ingestion.

Estrace, 17-beta estradiol, is not obtained from horse urine, seems to be more effective at a lower dose than Premarin, tends to cause fewer adverse effects, and is chosen by women patients over other

The Period of Sex Steroid Experimentation

estrogenic steroids when they are given a choice. Estrace has been available for years and is approved for osteoporosis therapy, yet inexplicably physicians prescribe Premarin more often. Even many elderly women physicians, who may have osteoporosis themselves, take Premarin.

When estrogenic steroids first became available for clinical use to treat postmenopausal osteoporosis and other conditions, some of the same difficulties that had been experienced in the early clinical use of testosterone and anabolic-androgenic steroids occurred again. The development of estrogenic steroids for clinical use had preceded the laboratory tests that would assist physicians in determining the proper dosage for these sex steroids. In effect, postmenopausal women in the 1960s and 1970s who were treated with these sex steroids were subjects of experimentation.

Let us not forget the younger women who effectively took part in another great medical experiment by taking oral contraceptives for years and years. What if taking oral contraceptives turns out to cause osteoporosis in later life by reducing the younger woman's peak bone mineral density?

My own opinion is that anything that reduces the ovarian production of testosterone may cause a decreased bone mineral density. Suppression of ovarian function, as is produced by certain types of birth control pills, may do just that. However, it may take decades of research to uncover the consequences of this great American experiment.

The dosages of estrogenic steroid therapy prescribed in the early years were so high as to cause very significant adverse effects in many women, including strokes, thrombophlebitis (blood clots), hypertension, major mood swings, personality changes, body fat gain, fluid retention, breast swelling, tenderness and perhaps breast cancer. It is tragic but undeniable that the dosages of these steroids prescribed by some of the nation's physicians early on did harm and even kill some women. The medical profession had no way to learn about estrogenic sex steroid replacement except by trial and error on real patients, especially as most areas of medical technology still lagged far behind the production of prescription drugs, which were proliferating rapidly.

When it became clear by the 1970s that harm was being done by these large doses, physicians became much less likely to prescribe estrogenic steroids at all for postmenopausal women. Medical students and residents were misled by incomplete and incorrect information about the early experimentation on American women. Today younger physicians who attempt to encourage postmenopausal women (who may have experienced major adverse effects to the higher doses of years ago) to restart sex steroid replacement therapy confront a major credibility problem.

For instance, it is not uncommon for a 70 to 75-year-old woman with severe osteoporosis to report that her doctor 25 years ago told her never to take an estrogen product again. Perhaps she suffered a major adverse effect when much higher doses of these steroids were prescribed. But the window of opportunity to help this woman, even in the face of already crippling osteoporosis, has probably been lost.

Older women who have experienced or heard of the problems caused by estrogenic steroids in high doses may tend to distrust younger physicians on the topic of sex steroid replacement and refuse appropriate preventive medical therapy. The consequences are poorer health and a greater economic burden on taxpayers — neither of which anyone wants.

Summary

In this chapter, the early history of sex steroid experimentation has been discussed, in terms of both scientific research and medical dogma. Some of the early findings are now buried in decades-old medical journals and medical textbooks, for reasons that have little scientific basis. This chapter has further defined the osteoporosis epidemic and its historical causative factors. This chapter, as well as the next chapters, describes some of the medical establishment's mistakes which helped to create such a bizarre epidemic. This chapter has also pointed to the fact that osteoporosis is an ever-draining disease, both financially and socially, on the American public. But it has a solution and cure.

Chapter 3

The Period of False Dogma

As I have argued already, missteps and ill-founded beliefs on the part of the medical establishment are in large part responsible for the prevalence of osteoporosis today. Although some evidence to this effect was presented in Chapter 2 in the course of describing the history of sex steroid experimentation, more examples will be presented and discussed in this chapter. The previous chapter laid the foundation for an understanding of where some of the ideas examined in this chapter came from. Misinformation rooted in the period of experimentation is the real culprit behind the current osteoporosis epidemic in the United States.

It was taught, for example, that providing supplemental dietary calcium for a postmenopausal woman may cause kidney stones, especially if the calcium supplementation is in the form of calcium bicarbonate. Therefore, such a practice was discouraged.

Today, medical science has proven that calcium supplementation is a safe and effective ingredient for fighting osteoporosis, although in most cases it cannot, in and of itself, prevent or treat osteoporosis. The calcium must get into the bone cell by osteoblast stimulation; once the osteoblast is stimulated, calcium can then be utilized in a normal manner to increase or maintain bone mineral density. But, for decades, medical students and physicians were taught otherwise.

It was also taught that the policies regarding estrogenic steroid replacement were confusing, and as a result many physicians avoided replacing these sex steroids in postmenopausal women entirely. Today, we know that the proper estrogenic steroid therapy is a major element in the appropriate treatment of postmenopausal osteoporosis and other postmenopausal conditions.

During the era of clinical experimentation various "medical authorities" influenced the opinions of textbook writers, who in turn influenced medical students and practicing physicians. The information the latter group received was based on incomplete research and was unreliable, but it was taught strictly as fact. And most physicians decided it was safer (for themselves) to accept what they were taught and to avoid prescribing any sex steroid therapy for postmenopausal women.

Similarly it was taught that testosterone and anabolic-androgenic steroid replacement had no role in women patients. In fact, this form of sex steroid therapy had been in scientific disrepute for so long that the mere mention of such a practice would infuriate many physicians. The general antipathy toward prescribing these steroids for women patients was extremely profound.

Testosterone and anabolic-androgenic steroids were considered nothing more than placebos by many physicians, and those who treated patients with them were viewed with suspicion. These drugs became the forgotten sex steroids for the treatment of menopausal osteoporosis and other postmenopausal conditions. A standard medical text, *Harrison's Principles of Internal Medicine*, eighth edition (1977), stated, "So-called anabolic steroids are weak androgens, and there is no advantage of their use in women in view of their masculinizing properties. There is also no proved advantage to combinations of estrogens and androgens." In fact testosterone and anabolic-androgenic steroids, with and without estrogenic steroids, had been shown in several scientific publications to have positive effects on menopausal osteoporosis and other postmenopausal conditions.

Given the prevalence of such miscommunication and indecisiveness about the use of anabolic-androgenic steroids, it is not surprising that osteoporosis has reached epidemic proportions in America and that recent attempts to educate postmenopausal women about the necessity to consider taking sex steroid replacement have frequently met stubborn resistance. Promotion of decades of medical misinformation has serious consequences.

Osteoporosis has killed many American women and crippled countless others to the point that they cannot walk without assistance; in many cases their skeletons have crumbled so greatly that they are in chronic pain and cannot function any longer. Moreover, there are currently millions of American women on the mere brink of a hip fracture that will place them in a nursing home — and most don't even know it.

Swayed by incomplete information that was later recounted as fact in textbooks, too many medical authorities have tried to make the practice of medicine conform to the way they *want* it practiced. Consequences of this tendency are reflected in the record-setting malpractice awards of 1995. Like Procrustes, stretching or hacking his victims to fit his iron bed, modern medicine has ignored the interests of its patients in its determination to mold the facts into compliance with a preconceived idea. If we want to conquer osteoporosis, we must be open-minded enough to do whatever actually works.

All foods, vitamins, minerals, drugs, sex steroids and polypeptide hormones are molecules. There is no doubt that if one supplies the human body with the proper molecules, it will tend to use them in the proper way. And for postmenopausal women their molecular question may be very simple: Have I taken the correct sex steroids today?

Chapter 4

The Proper Diagnosis, Treatment, Reversal and Cure of Osteoporosis

Introduction

The major key for reversing osteoporosis in the usual case for perimenopausal or postmenopausal women lies with the replacement of the sex steroids that the ovaries formerly produced. To mimic through therapy the quantities and types of sex steroids produced by the ovaries seems so natural and so simple, and it is the solution so desperately needed. But there may be some trial and error involved with each woman; after all, the quantities of these sex steroids vary widely in normal women. The previous chapters have attempted to explain why the medical establishment has opposed this obvious concept so strongly.

This book is not intended to embrace everything ever published on osteoporosis or to promote the usual means of managing the disease. There are dozens of such books already published which are not helping people. Neither are this book and this chapter intended to promote herbs and such as therapy for this disease, for others have published anti-establishment books of this nature without a strong scientific basis. This text is different in that it is based on scientific facts and concepts which will stand the test of time.

My method of practice has always been patient-oriented. If my method is correct and the medical establishment is wrong, then I won't practice their way. If I treat and cure osteoporosis and soothe other postmenopausal conditions like my forefathers in medicine intended, then I will do it for the sake of my patients. It may buck the "standard of care" in medicine, at times.

But the sad fact is that many physicians practice medicine to make money and protect the brotherhood of the medical establishment because they are either too afraid to go up against it or are too involved with making money. The medical establishment is losing respect daily because of these traits. Any time doctors put the approval of the establishment ahead of the individuals they serve or treat, the profession begins to have problems.

Basic Principles of Bone Metabolism

Historically, much of the medical emphasis on osteoporosis has focused on prevention, because reversing or curing it seemed so unlikely. But understanding the basic principles of bone metabolism, both before and after the menopause, may provide some insights as to how to combat postmenopausal osteoporosis with a variety of medications.

Normal bone metabolism consists of the processes of bone formation and bone resorption (dissolving or remodeling). These processes are regulated to a great degree by various polypeptide hormones, sex steroid hormones, minerals, and other molecular and environmental factors. Two basic bone cell types are regulated by these parameters: osteoblasts (bone formers) and osteoclasts (bone resorpters). Normal bone metabolism keeps a homeostasis or equilibrium

Proper Diagnosis, Treatment, Reversal and Cure

Figure 1: Simplified Basic Bone Metabolism

A. *osteoblast*
(incorporates blood calcium and other minerals into bone matrix)

Some osteoblast stimulators
anabolic-androgenic steroids
growth hormone
growth factors
vitamin D
weight bearing exercise
fluoride
tamoxifen (Nolvadex)
melatonin (?)

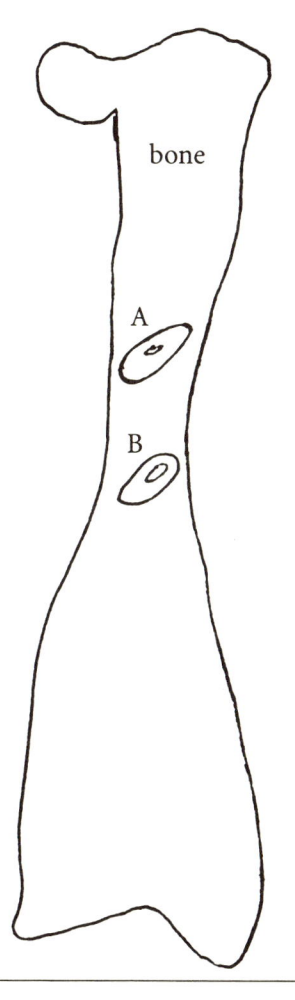

B. *osteoclast*
(dissolves bone, releasing calcium into bloodstream)

Some osteoclast inhibitors
estrogenic steroids
parathyroid hormone
calcitonin
bisphosphonates

between these two cells which have opposing functions as shown in Figure 1. Normal bone metabolism is slow, but it is steady; thus it takes several weeks for bone fractures to heal but only days for skin lacerations to heal by comparison.

Men normally have much stronger bones and a much higher bone mineral density than women do throughout life because of the higher levels of testosterone and anabolic-androgenic steroid production in men. From this fact alone, it would seem obvious that to reverse the osteoporosis process, that androgens would play the dominant role.

Recent studies have clearly shown that perimenopausal women may begin to have a reduction in the ovarian production of the three classes of sex steroids. This may result in a silent loss of bone mineral density due to diminished osteoblast activity and enhanced osteoclast activity. In other words, as the levels of sex steroids begin to diminish, there is a net dissolving of bone structure and calcium loss compared to the rate of bone formation and calcium incorporation. Over the years, this process can be a precursor for osteoporosis as women approach menopause proper.

Ovarian production of testosterone and other androgens takes place within the stromal tissue cells. These androgens may begin to diminish prior to the menopause proper, in a phenomenon some authors refer to as "andropause." Another source of androgens for women is the adrenal glands. For most women, approximately 85 percent of the body's testosterone is believed to be produced by the ovaries, while the adrenal glands contribute about 15 percent. However, there has been much controversy over the quantities of testosterone produced by the ovaries and the adrenal glands, with some researchers identifying the adrenal glands as the major producers of testosterone.

Although the testosterone produced in a woman's body probably does average about 85 percent ovarian and 15 percent adrenal, any given woman may vary from these percentages. When a woman enters andropause the major source of testosterone production diminishes, and it is unlikely that the adrenal glands can increase their production to make up the difference; therefore, testosterone levels may diminish for the remainder of her life. It follows, then, that if a woman becomes androgen deficient, she will have a concomitant major decrease in osteoblast functioning. Less serum calcium and other minerals will be incorporated normally into the bone matrix; this

Proper Diagnosis, Treatment, Reversal and Cure

phenomenon causes lower bone mineral density. Since andropause may occur prior to the menopause proper, it may help explain why more than 50 percent of all white women over the age of 45 years already have some degree of osteoporosis.

Ovarian estrogenic and progesterogenic steroids are made in the oocytes (eggs). There is a finite number of ovarian eggs which a woman will ever possess; it is determined early in fetal life and varies from woman to woman. The traditional view of the menopause describes it as essentially a matter of running out of eggs to ovulate and to produce sex steroids. Once the eggs have been ovulated over the decades and subsequently have been either fertilized or discarded through menses, no more eggs exist. Therefore, there will be no more eggs available to produce the sex steroids estrogen and progesterone, and menses will stop. The tissue that surrounds the ovarian eggs contains the stromal cells. Normally, a small amount of the progesterone made by the ovarian eggs is converted by the stromal cells to androgens. At the menopause proper, the human ovaries lose the capacity to manufacture and intraconvert all three of the sex steroid classes. Therefore, the postmenopausal woman becomes deficient in all three classes of sex steroids.

When the levels of estrogenic steroids diminish in a woman's body, so usually does the inhibition of the osteoclast. Estrogens are strong inhibitors of osteoclast functioning. Once the osteoclast becomes less inhibited, it dissolves bone structure at a faster pace than it would otherwise. This upsets the normal bone balance between the osteoblast and the osteoclast, giving rise to a loss of calcium from the bones and a lower bone mineral density and bone strength.

Thus it becomes very apparent that the basic bone metabolism can become greatly out of balance during the perimenopausal and postmenopausal years. With less sex steroid production, there is less bone structure formation and more bone structure dissolving, day by day, with osteoporosis the result.

Therefore, methods to rebalance the normal bone metabolism should focus both on factors which stimulate the osteoblast and on factors which inhibit the osteoclast. Appropriate sex steroid replacement can perform the needed functions. The specifics about the proper sex steroid replacement which both stimulates the osteoblast and inhibits the osteoclast will be discussed later in this chapter.

Diagnosis and Longitudinal Follow-Up

Proper diagnostic testing must be the cornerstone for the baseline study of bone mineral density and diagnosis of osteoporosis, and periodic retesting is important to determine whether or not a particular therapy is having the desired effects. To invoke a very common analogy, prescribing "standard" sex steroid therapy for osteoporosis without a definitive bone mineral density text and follow-up testing would be like treating a diabetic with a "standard" dose of insulin without ever measuring baseline and subsequent blood sugars! Or, for a patient with hypothyroidism, prescribing a "standard" dose of thyroid hormone for therapy and never measuring subsequent thyroid levels.

Nonetheless, many physicians as of this writing are not obtaining bone mineral density tests for their postmenopausal patients! What is perhaps even more absurd is that for many physicians, today's standard of care for osteoporosis is to prescribe a "standard" dose of Premarin and never obtain bone mineral studies before or after sex steroid therapy.

The most accurate and safest bone mineral density testing machine currently available for the diagnosis and longitudinal follow-up for osteoporosis is the dual-energy X-ray absorptiometer (DEXA), a device approved for use by the FDA in the late 1980s. This author had the first DEXA machine in the state of Florida in 1990. The DEXA machine is now available in almost all areas of the country.

Today's medical, osteopathic, podiatric, chiropractic, dental, surgical and psychiatric physicians who are treating perimenopausal and postmenopausal women should prescribe a bone mineral density study for these women. But by and large they do not—and often, these physicians see signs of osteoporosis but remain silent about it. A recent study strongly suggests that prescribing a DEXA scan for these women is a cost-effective use of health care monies. To ignore bone mineral density studies, at this point in time, in this huge group of women, is rapidly becoming tantamount to malpractice. Any malpractice attorney who examined the medical records of postmenopausal white women who have sustained hip fractures could easily determine whether a physician had documentation that bone density studies and sex steroid replacement therapy had been discussed with the patient.

Postmenopausal osteoporosis is a disease that crosses the boundaries between several distinct medical disciplines. But physicians in all of these disciplines have been exceedingly slow to prescribe the DEXA scans for their perimenopausal and postmenopausal women.

As an example of this phenomenon, when I served as a cardiovascular rehabilitation physician in a large city in Florida, I observed that during the calendar year of 1993, not a single postmenopausal white woman who was referred for cardiac rehabilitation was even prescribed sex steroid therapy, much less a DEXA scan. These women had already sustained a myocardial infarction, percutaneous transluminal angioplasty (PCTA) or coronary artery bypass surgery. Especially considering the cardioprotective benefits of estrogens, this type of "community standard of care" strikes me as being tantamount to malpractice.

The days of guesswork are essentially over now that the DEXA machines are widely available to help direct the diagnosis and treatment of osteoporosis. Doctors are no longer "shooting from the hip," blindly prescribing some arbitrary dose of a sex steroid without periodic bone mineral density studies to determine the effect, or lack of effect, that therapy is having on any given woman patient. Physicians who continue refusing to consider osteoporosis as a disease or to order DEXA scans for their perimenopausal and postmenopausal women may soon find themselves convinced by a medical malpractice suit or two.

With regards to osteoporosis testing, this author has exclusively used the DEXA scanner, and for good reasons. But various hospitals and

Osteoporosis

other osteoporosis centers have continued to use other types of equipment.

One machine which is still used, but is to a lessening degree, is the quantitative computer tomography (QCT) machine. Although QCT is grossly inferior to DEXA testing, and repeated QCT scans can be dangerous to the patient from repeated X-ray exposure, a few hospitals and clinics are still conducting QCT studies on patients for the diagnosis and follow-up of osteoporosis.

Duel-energy X-ray absorptiometry (DEXA) overcomes the large errors of precision, reproducibility and accuracy of the older quantitative computer tomography (QCT) approach of measuring bone mineral density of the spine. The large percentage of error of QCT prevents its use for monitoring small changes in bone density over time, and there is up to a 20 percent variance among different QCT machines' data.

The radiation dose of DEXA is 250–1000 times smaller, and DEXA offers bone density measurement of the femur necks (hips), the site of the most debilitating osteoporotic fractures, whereas QCT is limited to the spine. The Technology Assessment Group of the American Medicine Association has reviewed DEXA positively, and it is reimbursed by Medicare.

Currently, QCT scans are no longer used by experts in osteoporosis, or by leading university hospitals for either research or clinical management. Even the radiologists who developed the older QCT approach at the University of California–San Francisco now use DEXA for clinical management. Moreover, the research clinical trials for osteoporosis in the United States and throughout the world use DEXA.

The DEXA test is a rapid scan and the cost to the patient is relatively low. Patients do not have to endure a 20-minute procedure as with QCT. The output from DEXA is based on reference data collected from thousands of normal patients, both male and female.

Only about 200 female patients are used for QCT normals, and the normal values vary with the type of QCT scanner and calibration phantom. In contrast, DEXA results are directly comparable to those

Proper Diagnosis, Treatment, Reversal and Cure

produced anywhere in the world at thousands of leading osteoporosis centers.

It should be obvious that the DEXA machine is the only type of technology today to use for the diagnosis and follow-up tests required for the proper management of osteoporosis. But what good is modern technology when physicians refuse to use it because of ignorance, apathy or hospital politics? Hospital politics is a particularly nasty business, as a letter sent out in 1994 by the administration of a local hospital to physicians in my area demonstrates. This letter referred to doctors who operate osteoporosis screening clinics as "entrepreneurs" and incorrectly described the QCT test as state-of-the-art. (The hospital, of course, had the QCT scanner and the clinics, including mine, used DEXA.)

One fact continues to be very disturbing in this matter. In my medical files I have case after case of patients with normal bone mineral density in the lumbar spine yet very osteoporotic hips. These are cases which QCT would have missed entirely over and over again. And of course these are not simply "cases"; they are women's lives.

The choice for the patient is to insist on a bone mineral density scan using DEXA for both the definitive diagnosis and longitudinal studies. All other tests are inferior, inaccurate and even dangerous because of their higher radiation exposure. Get a DEXA scan; insist on it. Also, insist on periodic rescanning to determine whether or not your prescribed therapy is working.

Calcium Supplementation

Calcium supplementation is also very important for the proper therapy for osteoporosis prevention and treatment. Calcium, in and of itself, will not actually treat, reverse or cure osteoporosis, but once the osteoblast (bone structure former) is stimulated, the calcium can enter the bone matrix structure in a normal fashion.

The type of calcium supplement matters somewhat. The two

major questions one needs to ask are very simple: Is the calcium supplement going to get into my bones? and What will be the cost of such a supplement? Studies have indicated that calcium carbonate is perhaps the most absorbed type of calcium, and it comes in a variety of forms.

Remember, it is the elemental calcium which counts, not the total milligrams of the calcium tablet. Calcium may be complexed with other anions, such as phosphate or citrate. Among the popular calcium supplements, generic calcium carbonate is the best buy and is therefore recommended. Whatever type of calcium supplement is chosen, the patient should take from 1000 to 1500 milligrams of elemental calcium daily.

Drugs for Osteoporosis Prevention and Treatment

Over the decades a number of drugs have been used for the treatment of osteoporosis. Some of these drugs have been indicated and approved for the treatment of osteoporosis by the FDA. One class of drugs, androgens, were approved by the FDA for treatment of osteoporosis for decades, but no longer. However, androgens have still been used successfully. The drugs approved by the FDA for treatment of osteoporosis are listed in Table 2.

The only drugs which have ever been approved by the FDA and have been significant stimulators of the osteoblast are the androgen sex steroids. All of the other FDA-approved drugs are essentially only osteoclast inhibitors. In the usual sense of preventing osteoporosis, it may be that one or more osteoclast inhibitors are helpful, but once significant osteoporosis is diagnosed, an osteoblast-stimulating androgen should be considered.

For most women who already have been diagnosed with osteoporosis, the combination of an estrogenic steroid and an anabolic-androgenic steroid should reverse the bone mineral density losses. The American pioneer who studied the effects of combined estrogen-

Table 2: FDA-Approved Drugs for Osteoporosis Therapy

Drug Name	Class	Mechanism	Approval
Depotestosterone	androgen	osteoblast stimulator	1960s*
Dianabol	androgen	osteoblast stimulator	1960s*
Deca-Durabolin	androgen	osteoblast stimulator	1960s*
Winstrol	androgen	osteoblast stimulator	1960s*
Estratest	combination androgen-estrogen	combination osteoblast stimulator-osteoclast inhibitor	1960s*
Premarin	estrogen	osteoclast inhibitor	1960s
Estrace	estrogen	osteoclast inhibitor	1980s
Ogen	estrogen	osteoclast inhibitor	1970s
Calcimar	calcitonin	osteoclast inhibitor	1980s
Miacalcin	calcitonin	osteoclast inhibitor	1995
Fosamax	bisphosphonate	osteoclast inhibitor	1995

*FDA approval dropped for osteoporosis indication in 1980s

---

androgen therapy in women for over 50 years was Dr. Robert Greenblatt. He stated in 1987, in one of his last publications prior to his death, and while still fighting the pressures of the medical establishment as he had done for decades, that

> Androgens are psychotropic drugs, participating in both physiologic and psychologic components of sexual behavior. They modulate the neurohumors of the brain and influence affective behavior. Androgens in nonvirilizing doses complement estrogens, are synergistic rather than contraphysiologic, and may be employed effectively by most women administered alone or in combination with an estrogen. The menopausal woman who has failed to experience the benefits of estrogen

replacement should be offered a trial of estrogen-androgen combination. Androgens are helpful in many gynecologic and nongynecologic disorders. Their use has not been exploited fully [*Obstetrics & Gynecology of North America* (1987)].

Traditionally, estrogenic steroids have been the primary choice by the medical establishment for sex steroid therapy in women for treating the symptoms and illnesses associated with the menopause. Many women, however, continue predictably to experience menopausal symptoms even with estrogen monotherapy. It really should be no surprise. The ovary makes three classes of sex steroids, and when it stops, why give back only one class and expect good results?

For some women estrogen monotherapy seems to work quite well, until one considers the osteoporosis process, and on that front estrogen monotherapy often predictably fails. What physician really knows his woman patient, these days, well enough to ask the right questions about her menopausal state? Too many doctors just seem to hope their women patients won't complain much — and if they do complain of depression, hot flashes, mood swings and loss of sex drive, they tend to refer them to psychiatrists, the only result of which is to make their perimenopausal and postmenopausal patients look foolish.

Combination estrogen-androgen therapy has been medically belittled long enough. Each of these classes of sex steroids has important physiological and psychological roles. They have great value, when used properly in perimenopausal and postmenopausal women. Estrogen-androgen therapy is the cornerstone therapy for reversing and curing the osteoporosis condition, as well as several other conditions of the postmenopausal years. Estrogens and androgens work together; they do not somehow oppose each other as many physicians still believe.

Some of the beneficial effects that the proper estrogen-androgen therapy can offer postmenopausal women, without virilizing effects, are listed in Table 3.

Table 3: Benefits of Proper Estrogen-Androgen Therapy in Postmenopausal Women

Estrogen Effect	Androgen Effect
protects cardiovascular system	maintains lean body mass
maintains vaginal compliance	maintains or enhances libido
maintains vaginal secretions	reduces memory loss
reduces wrinkling	reduces hot flashes
reduces memory loss	increases energy level
reduces hot flashes	stimulates osteoblasts
reduces depression	enhances adherence to therapy
maintains scalp hair quality	enhances quality of life
inhibits osteoclasts	enhances longevity
reduces cholesterol levels	delays aspects of aging
enhances quality of life	
enhances longevity	
delays aspects of aging	

Androgens (testosterone and anabolic-androgenic steroids) are the most important agents in the reversal of osteoporosis because they provide the most efficient way to stimulate the osteoblasts. A number of synthetic androgens have been shown to increase bone mineral density, but the ones with a high therapeutic index, such as Winstrol and Deca-Durabolin, have been shown to stimulate the osteoblast with the greatest margin of safety. Winstrol (stanolozol) has been shown to stimulate the osteoblasts directly, and the increased bone mineral density associated with Winstrol therapy in men and women restores normal bone metabolism, according to the recent methods to study bone biopsies.

In short, it has been scientifically proven that androgens, like Winstrol, can reverse and even cure major deficits in bone mineral density without virilizing effects. Winstrol is a very potent osteoblast stimulator, even in low doses.

Osteoporosis

The use of androgens in women has waxed and waned over the decades but appears to be gaining respect in the 1990s. A recent scientific symposium was held in May 1995 in San Francisco, California, on the "Emerging Role of Androgens in Menopausal Treatment." Several scientific lectures were given by specialists from across the country. Some of the salient points which were made are listed below.

• Women who use sex steroid replacement (combination estrogen-androgen) therapy in menopause lead better lives, as judged by most quality-of-life measures, and live longer as well. Sex steroid replacement therapy should be provided for all women who desire it, and should be continued indefinitely. Many women can expect to live nearly half of their lifespan suffering from the sequelae of ovarian involution. Menopause should be considered as a continuum rather than a passage.

• Androgens may be used to improve quality of life without detracting from the cardiovascular benefits of estrogenic steroid replacement. Androgens have a growing role in menopause therapy when combined with estrogenic steroids, and they appear to be both safe and beneficial.

• Treatment with combined estrogenic and androgenic steroids can increase bone mineral density more than estrogenic steroids alone and relieve somatic symptoms of menopause better than estrogen alone. Addition of an androgenic steroid to the replacement therapy has a positive effect on osteoblast activity, which is not seen with estrogenic steroids.

• By correlating perceived distress from menopausal symptoms with sexual drive, the physician can offer treatment and improve the potential for the patient's adherence to therapy for the other aspects of menopause, by utilizing combined estrogenic and androgenic steroids. Estrogen-androgen therapy improves energy and mood in menopausal women. Testosterone and anabolic-androgenic steroids appear to be responsible for sexual drive in women, and sexual drive has been shown to increase adherence to therapy in some women after estrogen-androgen replacement.

Proper Diagnosis, Treatment, Reversal and Cure

• Progesterogenic steroids can be added to the treatment regimen to help reduce the small risk of uterine cancer.

Estrogen-androgen combination therapy is finally emerging as the correct method to treat many of the conditions associated with the postmenopausal years, including osteoporosis. The advent of the DEXA machine will help to prove what a few medical pioneers knew decades ago. The DEXA machine gives medical science a major objective measurement which it has never really had before. As in many areas of medicine, further research is needed to refine treatment regimens. More researchers are headed in the correct direction to reverse or perhaps cure osteoporosis by attempting to mimic the normally functioning ovaries. This author's work toward that goal has resulted thus far in two research papers that indicate remarkable results in reversing and curing major deficits in bone mineral density. Of course, no one can promise that fractures can be reversed or that lost height can be reestablished, but the bone mineral density can be returned to the normal range so that future fractures are much less likely to occur.

A summary of these two studies will be presented below. We began the studies in 1990 when the medical profession tended to ostracize those who prescribed androgens for women. We had the DEXA machine and I was ready to study the effects of estrogen-androgen combination therapy on a small number of women volunteers. I wanted to apply my theory that the addition of a cyclical low-dose androgen to an existing estrogen therapy could safely reverse major deficits in bone mineral density.

In our study, published in 1992, we studied a select group of three women. They were all members of our sports and preventive medicine clinic and worked out on a regular basis. They were all physically fit, attractive, married and active. All three women had undergone the surgical menopause in years past, but had taken Premarin continuously until they were studied in our osteoporosis center. We evaluated their bone mineral densities with the DEXA machine and found that all three were osteoporotic and had lost an average of at least 30 percent of their bone densities. We performed a complete physical exam, blood work studies and a graded exercise stress test before and after the study. These women also habitually took calcium and a multivitamin daily prior to and during the study. In short, these women were doing everything correctly, according to the standard of care adopted by the medical establishment. They were chosen for the reason that they would be the ideal group to show that truer mimicking of the normal ovarian function could reverse major bone mineral density loss. We changed only their sex steroid replacement therapy to include 5 mg of Provera (progesterogenic steroid) and 2mg of Winstrol (anabolic-androgenic steroid) for ten calendar days each month. After six months, the women averaged an increase in bone mineral density of 14.1%, a reduction in percentage body fat of 8.0 percent and a stable body weight. They all reported an increased self-esteem, energy level and libido.

There were no adverse effects reported by them or found in the physical exam or repeat blood evaluations. Contrary to the popular beliefs of that time that androgen therapy would lower the desirable high density cholesterol, we found that this sex steroid therapy actually raised this value slightly. This pilot study indicated that triple sex steroid replacement therapy effectively, safely and inexpensively reverses major deficits in bone mineral density in postmenopausal women who have not adequately responded to estrogenic steroid replacement alone.

In a second study published in 1994, we studied six postmenopausal women who either had not been treated with sex steroids or who had been treated with Premarin and Provera or bisphosphonate therapy prior to being studied. All six women were found to be osteoporotic and had lost an average of 30 percent of their bone mineral densities, as determined by DEXA testing. We discontinued their previous therapy and placed them on a combined estrogen-androgen regimen. Each woman was placed on Estrace (1mg/day) and Winstrol (2mg/day for only ten days each month). After six months, increases in bone mineral density averaged 19.1 percent. Two women continued this therapy for 12 months, which resulted in an average bone mineral density of 28 percent, which placed them back into the normal range for age-matched women. There were no virilizing effects or bone fractures noted during the treatment period. This small study indicated that major deficits in bone mineral density could be reversed safely and inexpensively by this form of sex steroid therapy over a short period of time.

We postulated that the osteoblasts in the usual case of postmenopausal osteoporosis were somewhat dormant and that we could stimulate these cells with a short burst of Winstrol for ten days on a low-dose schedule. The normal ovarian production of androgens is greatest for about ten days each month, just before and just after ovulation. We also postulated that this cyclical low-dose regimen would reduce any tolerance to the Winstrol; therefore, we could give the same low-dose, short burst over and over again to restimulate the osteoblasts. Moreover, we postulated that once the osteoblasts were stimulated each month, they would go about their normal function, taking in calcium and minerals to create a normal, strong bone structure. We chose Winstrol because of its high therapeutic index and because it had been scientifically shown to produce what bone biopsies had proven to be normal bone formation.

In summary, I believe that the appropriate regimen of sex steroid replacement is paramount in reversing major deficits in bone mineral density. I strongly recommend that the sex steroid replacement consist of Estrace and cyclical Winstrol. For most women, Estrace doses should be between 0.5mg and 1.0mg daily and Winstrol should be from 2mg to 4mg daily for about ten days each month. If the risk of uterine cancer is a worry, a progesterogenic steroid may be added to the regimen.

Discussion

Isn't Winstrol (stanozolol) the anabolic-androgenic steroid that Ben Johnson, who ran the world's fastest time ever in the 100-meter dash in the 1988 Olympic Games, took and tested positive

Osteoporosis

for? Yes, it is. Isn't Winstrol one of the most popular anabolic-androgenic steroids used by strength athletes in a variety of sports? Yes, it is.

So, the drug that helped a man run the fastest 100-meter time ever recorded, and by a good margin, helps reverse and perhaps even cure osteoporosis? Yes. How can a drug which helps athletes build such imposingly muscular bodies be of any value in the treatment of osteoporosis? The answer is that Winstrol's osteoblast stimulating characteristic can be realized at very low doses. In comparison to the huge amounts necessary to enhance athletic performance and produce imposingly muscular bodies, it takes very little of the steroid to stimulate the osteoblasts.

For most people, two cups of coffee daily are safe, but how about 200 cups of coffee daily? Such an intake would be lethal for many. For most people, two aspirins daily are safe, but how about 200 aspirins daily? Lethal for most. For most people, two ibuprofen tablets a day are safe, but how about 200 ibuprofen tablets daily? Again, lethal for most. And to further the point, for most people, two daily drinks of ethanol are safe, but how about 200 drinks daily? Such a dose would be lethal. By the same token, for a postmenopausal woman, 2 to 4 milligrams of Winstrol daily for 10 days each month is a safe and recommended dose. Some athletes take 200 to 400 milligrams daily, and even then Winstrol is not likely to be lethal.

I have often faced criticism for prescribing Winstrol to my patients with osteoporosis, but the criticism has come from my colleagues and not my patients. The treatment strategy I have described works, and I find that ample reason to follow it.

The appropriate means of preventing, treating, reversing and perhaps even curing this disease has been known in America for several decades. Ever since the 1940s, some few women have received estrogen-androgen combination therapy for osteoporosis under prescription by a select few doctors. I have met some of these women, including some who were 80 years old or more. Many of these women were still sexually active and were found *not* to have osteoporosis by DEXA testing.

Proper Diagnosis, Treatment, Reversal and Cure

Winstrol was reviewed by osteoporosis therapy in the late 1960s by the National Academy of Sciences–National Research Council. Based on the findings of that study "and/or other information," the FDA classified Winstrol as "'probably' effective ... as adjunctive but not primary therapy in senile and postmenopausal osteoporosis," according to a 1971 package insert for Winstrol.

But what was taught to the medical profession about this class of sex steroids at this same time? Usually, the FDA is conservative about approving a drug for specific indications, so its endorsement would lead one to expect that Winstrol and other anabolic-androgenic steroids would have been used extensively to treat osteoporosis. Winstrol did have FDA approval, but this is what was taught:

> Anabolic-androgenic steroids are defined biologically as substances that stimulate male secondary sexual characteristics (masculinization). These are seen as clinical hirsutism (facial hair) and virilization of the female with amenorrhea (lack of menstrual periods), atrophy of the breasts and uterus, enlargement of the clitoris, deepening of the voice, acne, increased muscle mass, increased heterosexual drive, and receding hairline [*Harrison's Principles of Internal Medicine*, eighth edition, (1977)].

The above quote describes the conditions which tend to occur when a woman overproduces androgens or when much too large a dose is taken for too long a period of time. In effect, it describes the modern-day female bodybuilder who takes huge doses of these steroids for a long time. But these sex steroids when used in the proper doses are useful in a great number of clinical situations.

Other anabolic steroids also stimulate the osteoblast and are perhaps appropriate for osteoporosis therapy in women. The anabolic-androgenic steroid Dianabol (methandrostenolone) was also reviewed by the National Academy of Sciences–National Research Council and was classified as "'probably' effective as adjunctive therapy in senile and postmenopausal osteoporosis," according to a 1980 package insert for Dianabol.

Osteoporosis

In the 1980s the osteoporosis indication for anabolic-androgenic steroids was mysteriously removed from the approved indications in the *Physician's Desk Reference*. Not one single study ever published showed that this class of steroids did not treat osteoporosis, yet the FDA dropped the indication.

The effect was to again wipe this class of steroids off the scientific map. And this inexcusable error happened nearly a decade *before* the definitive osteoporosis scanner was even invented for clinical use.

But all along, and perhaps behind the scenes, NASA knew how to reverse osteoporosis that occurred in the space program. Prolonged space travel causes osteoporosis to develop in both men and women very quickly. Osteoporosis was one medical hurdle which had to be cleared in order to continue prolonged space flights, and to date, the only therapy which has worked has been treatment with anabolic-androgenic steroids. This type of therapy stimulates the osteoblasts even where exercise and other treatments have failed.

So what happened? Why did the FDA remove the osteoporosis indication from the package insert of Winstrol and the other anabolic-androgenic steroids? Was it because the FDA staff knew something that the rest of the medical scientists didn't? I for one find such a proposition impossible to believe. The FDA's action is a mystery.

False medical dogma and the overlooking of medical facts can be so counterproductive to the progress of medical science that the subsequent effects are nearly impossible to calculate. Such blunders usually result when true medical science comes into conflict with the "medical authorities" who represent the governing voice of the medical practice.

These vocal figures too often make premature conclusions about medical science with sometimes only a paucity of scientific studies published. This common thread appears again and again when the medical community makes major policy errors. Besides, what appointed "medical authority" ever discovered anything? They are frequently more involved with politicking themselves into positions of influence than with advancing medical science.

Proper Diagnosis, Treatment, Reversal and Cure

Misguided medical dogma and the erasure of the osteoporosis indication for the anabolic-androgenic steroids tied practicing physicians' hands to the point that postmenopausal women were practically doomed to suffer the consequences of postmenopausal osteoporosis. Prescribing no sex steroid therapy and no calcium supplementation was "state-of-the-art" in the 1970s and 1980s for many physicians. This practice would basically ensure that most white women would become osteoporotic.

Another medical practice contributed to the overall osteoporosis epidemic. The practice of performing the surgical menopause, through a hysterectomy and removal of the ovaries, became unnecessarily common. Sometimes it was performed for profit only. Many women who underwent the surgical menopause were never even started on sex steroid replacement therapy because of all of the prevailing misconceptions about its consequences. Meanwhile, thousands of women were losing bone mineral density and developing osteoporosis at relatively young ages. As the results of this surgery manifested themselves, these surgical physicians were not even treating the common menopausal conditions, as they could have done through sex steroid therapy. What was left was often a depressed young woman with no interet in sex.

For instance, a typical 35- to 40-year-old woman may have had a hysterectomy performed, perhaps even for birth control measures. If the surgeons removed the ovaries as well, and did not follow through with prescribing the important classes of sex steroids, the surgery would often have major consequences. Besides her subsequent mood swings, hot flashes, night sweats, depression, loss of energy and loss of sex drive, her vaginal mucosa, normally spongy and compliant, would become paper thin and easily torn during sexual intercourse. She would have little sexual desire, and when she did have intercourse, it was painful. Her husband typically would not understand, would become angry at her, and might even become unfaithful. She would subsequently be referred to a psychiatrist or a psychologist because her physician had become frustrated with the nature of her complaints. Her surgical physician might even feel that she was hysterical. Within

Osteoporosis

a few years her urinary bladder would tend to lose its elasticity and urinary frequency (small bladder syndrome) and urinary incontinence would result. She would eventually have to wear sanitary napkins because she could not control her bladder. The muscle and elastic tone of the pelvic region would deteriorate to the point where the vagina would prolapse and protrude forward. The lack of sex steroids can cause this scenario, and it has, over and over again. A woman with just such a story was 50 years old when she came to me for her osteoporosis scan.

Chapter 5

Alarming Physician Attitudes

In the previous chapters, I have tried to build the background for an understanding of elements which permitted osteoporosis to become an epidemic, and which still surround the treatment of the disease.

In a sense, I have been attempting to build a case for the reader to understand better the pressures that exist to push doctors away from the one treatment strategy that has actually worked to combat osteoporosis. In my medical practice I have seen countless postmenopausal women patients who were being treated by a variety of physicians who ignored the osteoporosis condition.

The following accounts involve real case studies and personal professional experiences. The information extracted from them is anecdotal, but I feel these incidents are interesting and often enlightening. Many of the questions, even the ones brought up by physicians, are commonly encountered, and I hope that readers may gain a deeper understanding of the osteoporosis epidemic, perhaps even of their own condition, by reading this chapter.

My practice involved lecturing to physicians, appearing on a regular weekly local television program entitled "Bones, Hormones and Hot Flashes," and diagnosing and treating osteoporosis in our clinics. I also usually spent about one day weekly calling on local physicians with one of my partners to market our osteoporosis clinic and explain my ideas on treating and reversing osteoporosis. On that day, in a sense, I was much like a typical pharmaceutical representative calling on physicians and other professionals. My calls on physicians in their offices often lasted over an hour and proved an enlightening experience for me and my partners who accompanied me. The attitudes we encountered made me step back and take a good, long look at the profession.

Below are summaries of several of these physician calls and confrontations as they relate to the osteoporosis epidemic.

Case 1: The Entrenched Gynecologist

In the fall of 1994 one of my partners and I called on one of our city's most prominent gynecologists. He was very influential in the county medical society. He was also my sister's gynecologist and had delivered her baby boy nearly ten years prior to our visit. After about 30 minutes of my presentation regarding our diagnostic and treatment center for osteoporosis and my concepts on estrogen-androgen therapy, he looked at me and said, "Young man, what you are telling me is against everything that I was ever taught on this subject. I am a very powerful physician in this community and I intend to notify the Board of Medicine regarding your radical treatment. By the way, I have never heard of this DEXA machine. Do any of the teaching institutions have the DEXA machine? Can you provide me with a listing of those teaching institutions that do? Otherwise, I'm going to report you to the Board of Medicine for radical medical treatment."

My partner and I were baffled, angry and incredulous. Thinking that he may have thought I was being dishonest with him, I jogged his recent memory about my role with the congressional reclassification

Alarming Physician Attitudes

of anabolic-androgenic steroids as controlled substances. He commented that this feat was something major to be proud of. I quickly replied that if he believed me about the importance of that work, then why would he not believe me on my osteoporosis work?

He claimed that he rarely referred a postmenopausal woman for a bone mineral density study, and when he did it was for the hospital-based QCT test. He seemed unwilling to consider anything else.

The only sex steroid which he would consider was Premarin therapy, and most of his postmenopausal patients were not on any sex steroid therapy. He refused to let us speak with his female gynecologist partners. My partner and I spent about 30 minutes watching a drove of menopausal women enter and leave his office. Some used walkers and some were in wheelchairs as a result of osteoporosis-related hip fractures.

In other words, this physician was still going to ignore the facts and treat his postmenopausal women patients the same old way that he always had. And, in effect, he would exert his power in the local medical community to ensure that many of the community's postmenopausal patients would suffer from debilitating osteoporosis. After calling on him, I was in mental turmoil, dismayed and disjointed.

Case 2: The Educated Gynecologist

In the fall of 1994 one of my partners and I called on a 40-year-old gynecologist in his office. He had just returned from a medical conference in which the roles of anabolic-androgenic steroids for the treatment of osteoporosis were presented. One of his physician friends spoke on the topic and quoted some of my work on estrogen-androgen therapy. He was aware of my Estrace-Winstrol regimen because his physician friend in southern California used this regimen for postmenopausal osteoporosis. I informed him that I knew his friend and that he had called me two years ago to discuss this treatment regimen. However, he told me that he was a big Premarin prescriber and that he used the QCT testing at the local hospital where he had privileges.

He told me that he felt uneasy about referring his postmenopausal women for a DEXA scan, even though he knew it was the definitive test, out of fear of being blackballed within the hospital's political scheme.

Case 3: The Herbal Internist

In the fall of 1994 one of my partners and I called on a female internal medicine physician who was from India. She was interested in the treatment of osteoporosis and she had a large number of elderly white women as patients. But she was "treating" osteoporosis without using DEXA scans and by placing her elderly women patients on one or more herbal products which she sold right out of her office.

The shelves of her office were loaded with bottles of herbs which made it look like a health food store. Of course, there was no way to judge whether or not any of these herbs had any effect on the osteoporosis condition of her patients, for she never even considered the need for bone mineral density studies. She seemed to be interested only in the profit motive. She also thought that the functioning human ovaries produced only estrogens and progesterones. I could see that my efforts to sway her were in vain.

Case 4: The Romantic Rheumatologist

In the winter of 1995 one of my partners and I had a business luncheon with a young, athletically fit woman rheumatologist. She showed a great deal of interest in my presentation and thought that many of her postmenopausal women could benefit from both the DEXA scan and estrogen-androgen therapy for osteoporosis. She worried,

Alarming Physician Attitudes

however, that altering a woman's mood and sexual drive could be too controversial for the local medical community. She told us that she depended on the support of the local medical community for her referrals and that she would feel uncomfortable about prescribing combined estrogen-androgen therapy. Even after I discussed with her the studies indicating that this sex steroid therapy might help her postmenopausal patients with rheumatoid arthritis as well, she still was reserved.

Her major dissenting remark was that she was worried about prescribing sex steroids which might enhance the sexual drive and orgasmic response of her women patients and how that would interact with her own feminist views.

Case 5: The Oblivious Orthopedist

During the fall of 1994 one of my partners and I called on a female orthopedic surgeon. She showed concern for the osteoporosis condition, but she was unaware of the DEXA testing. She was worried about developing osteoporosis herself, was postmenopausal, and was undergoing no sex steroid replacement. She felt that it was not her job to prescribe sex steroids for her elderly women patients. She had performed hip surgery on a few women in their late 30s who had contracted osteoporosis after undergoing the surgical menopause. Her office waiting area was swamped with postmenopausal women patients who were crippled by their condition. On occasion, she would refer a patient for a QCT test at the hospital. If she prescribed any sex steroid replacement at all for her postmenopausal patients, it was exclusively Premarin.

Case 6: The Contrary Cardiologist

During the summer of 1994 I spoke with a leading cardiologist in the medical community about sex steroid replacement and its role in reducing heart disease. We also discussed the osteoporosis condition in the community. I had confronted him in the lobby outside a convention room between lectures. I asked him why none of his women patients with heart disease, which I was monitoring during cardiac rehabilitation, were on estrogenic steroids for the cardioprotective effects of these steroids. He responded that prescribing sex steroids for his postmenopausal women patients was not his responsibility.

He appeared to believe that sex steroid prescription and follow-up were beneath him professionally. He told me that he felt insulted that I had even approached him about the topic.

Case 7: The Nasty Neurosurgeon

I met a neurosurgeon at a medical golf outing during the summer of 1994. He claimed that he was a major player in establishing Medicare reimbursement for various diagnostic tests in the state. He was very powerful in the local medical community. He seemed interested in my presentation from an educational point of view, but was very loyal to the local hospitals. He believed the DEXA test was some sort of gimmick, and he supported the QCT testing at the hospitals. He told me that he would use his influence to greatly reduce the Medicare reimbursement for DEXA. He viewed me as a direct threat to his surgical business. He has made his fortune, and continues to do so, from operating on osteoporotic patients to relieve their pain and suffering.

Case 8: The Fickle Family Physician

I had known this male physician for about two years, and he was a golfing buddy of mine. He was a proponent of preventive medicine and considered osteoporosis *the* disease of the twenty-first century, and in his residency training he had used DEXA testing for osteoporosis. He wrote a weekly column in the local paper about various aspects of preventive medicine. After my partners and I called on him on several occasions he referred many of his postmenopausal patients for DEXA scans. Then the local hospital, which subsidized the rent for his medical office, pressured him into using their QCT scan to keep himself in good stead with other referring physicians in the hospital.

Both his mother and father ultimately died from the sequelae of osteoporosis-related hip fractures. It was demoralizing to watch my friend succumb to the power of hospital politics, especially since he believed so much in preventive medicine and what our clinics were doing.

Case 9: The Educated Endocrinologist

In the fall of 1994 my partner and I called on a local endocrinologist who was current with his education regarding osteoporosis. During his residency training in endocrinology, he used DEXA testing to establish the diagnosis and follow-up bone mineral densities on his patients.

After his residency, he aligned with a hospital in our area which used QCT testing for the diagnosis and follow-up of osteoporosis. I confronted him on the issue of how he could use QCT over the DEXA scan, especially since he had trained with the DEXA machine. His face showed that he had an ethical conflict of interest and that he knew I knew it.

Then we discussed estrogen-androgen therapy for his postmenopausal patients with diagnosed osteoporosis. When I showed him some of our results, he was impressed and for a while referred many of his patients for DEXA scanning. The medical staff at the hospital convinced him otherwise, and he began again using QCT for the diagnosis and follow-up testing for osteoporosis. He was well aware that the DEXA testing was definitive and a safer test than QCT testing.

Case 10: *The Patient-Oriented Podiatrist*

I ran a half-marathon side by side with a male podiatrist in 1993. We had plenty of time to talk shop along the way. We also worked out together and talked shop on many occasions at a local health club. He believed in our clinic, the DEXA testing and my type of sex steroid therapy for osteoporosis.

We collaborated on a study with stress fractures, osteoporosis and estrogen-androgen therapy for both conditions. Our results should be published in the future.

Case 11: *The Objurgating Orthopedist*

In January 1995 I gave a grand rounds lecture at a local hospital on treating, reversing and curing osteoporosis. After the lecture an orthopedist scolded me and called my lecture too controversial. The hospital purchased a DEXA machine shortly after my lecture; then, on a local television program sponsored by the medical center associated with that hospital, this physician answered a call-in question regarding Winstrol therapy for osteoporosis. He replied, "We have an organization in the area that uses that anabolic steroid and under no circumstances would I suggest its use. They are male hormones and cause major side effects. Those are the steroids which are abused by athletes." Fortunately, I recognized the caller's voice and smoothed over the incident. But it is this type of ill-informed statement by a physician that can ruin another practice. I have often wondered how he would respond to the same kind of professional bad-mouthing if it were directed at him and his surgical techniques.

Case 12: *The Gullible Gynecologist*

In the winter of 1995 one of my partners and I called on a local gynecologist who was a golfing buddy of mine. After my presentation, he stated that he had never prescribed anabolic-androgenic steroids to any of his women patients. I quickly corrected him, for in fact he had many of his patients on Danocrine therapy for endometriosis. He looked shocked and questioned whether Danocrine was an anabolic-androgenic steroid.

We then got into a discussion about some of the adverse effects he had seen with the higher doses of Danocrine. He stated that Danocrine was not called an anabolic-androgenic steroid, but finally agreed that it acted like one.

Things like this happen in medicine. It may be hard to believe that a simple nomenclature change or mistake can influence a physician's knowledge or prescribing habits. But, it does; just ask the pharmaceutical industry. For instance, no two anabolic-androgenic steroids are structurally more alike than Winstrol and Danocrine. Winthrop Pharmaceutical Company developed both of these steroid molecules, Winstrol in the early 1960s and Danocrine over a decade later.

Winthrop marketed Winstrol as an anabolic steroid and later felt that Danocrine might be better accepted if it were classified an "antigonadotropic" steroid. Physicians accepted this artificial distinction in class nomenclature. Both Winstrol and Danocrine, however, are considered anabolic-androgenic steroids by the United States Olympic Committee's Drug Control Program because in large doses, they can enhance athletic performance in both male and female athletes.

Case 13: The Distinguished Dentist

My dentist and I usually talk about golf when I see him, but we have also discussed the osteoporosis condition. I got him to admit that he sees plenty of osteoporosis in his postmenopausal women when he takes X-rays of the jaw bone. This condition can cause loss of teeth as the jaw bone becomes porous and weak. He stated that he had never referred a patient for an osteoporosis evaluation because it was not his responsibility, even though osteoporosis is a major cause of tooth loss.

Discussion

This short chapter describes the recent attitudes of a variety of physicians in my local area when confronted directly about the osteoporosis epidemic. I did not include the attitudes of some of the supportive physicians, for I have indeed had many physicians who did refer patients to our osteoporosis clinics. And, working with these physicians, we have had good success in diagnosing and reversing this condition.

As concern about this disease continues to increase, it becomes apparent that perimenopausal and postmenopausal women may have to shop around for a physician who is current on osteoporosis and sex steroid replacement. After all, much of a woman's adult life will be postmenopausal. The appropriate sex steroid replacement may be the most important health care decision which she and her physician ever make.

Chapter 6

Contemporary Questions and Answers

The previous chapters have dealt with many of the issues which surround the osteoporosis epidemic. In the last chapter, my difficulties in attempting to confront and reeducate physicians on the various aspects of this problem revealed a variety of alarming attitudes. All major medical illnesses are made of many case studies with subtle differences which make for fertile ground for individual questions and answers. In this chapter, various questions which have come from my actual clinical experiences, local television show or lectures will be answered.

Question 1: Dr. Taylor, I am a 45-year-old woman who has been experiencing a premenstrual condition that seems to be worse than it was a few years ago. My sexual desire is low and I have very little energy most of the time. My gynecologist has recommended that I start on the birth control pill for these symptoms. My menstrual periods are still fairly regular, but I have fewer days of bleeding. What do you think about this?

Answer: Some physicians are prescribing birth control pills for women with perimenopausal symptoms similar to yours. Many women that are your age are going through a gradual period of sex steroid production from the ovaries which are "sputtering." Sex steroid therapy, such as oral contraceptives, should be tailored to a woman's symptoms and conditions. With reduced sexual desire, I am inclined to believe that you are going through "andropause," which is a relative decline in androgen production from the stromal cells of the ovaries. Laboratory blood tests to determine sex steroid levels may or may not be important, primarily because the normal range values are very wide. I would recommend a bone mineral density test with the DEXA machine of both your spine and hips. If your sexual desire and energy level are not increased with the prescribed oral contraceptives, then I would consider addition of a cyclical low-dose anabolic-androgenic steroid, such as Winstrol, to your sex steroid therapy. I have had good results with adding 2mg of Winstrol daily for the first 10 days after the period starts each month.

Question 2: Dr. Taylor, I am a 48-year-old white woman who had her children years ago. My gynecologist prescribed monthly injections of Depo-Provera for the purpose of family planning and birth control. I have been taking the injections for nearly 8 years. My mother recently fractured one of her hips, is now in a nursing home, and has to use a walker to get around. Can you tell me if I should be worried about getting osteoporosis or not?

Answer: Postmenopausal osteoporosis in white women is so common that it is nearly impossible to determine all of the factors which may contribute to it. Certainly, osteoporosis tends to predispose along hereditary lines. But, of greater concern is your protracted use of progesterogenic steroids (Depo-Provera), with low androgen activity, for birth control measures. Basically, large monthly injections of a long-acting progesterogenic steroid may inhibit the production of the other ovarian sex steroids, namely androgens and estrogens, which play major roles in normal bone metabolism. The role of progesterogenic steroids on bone metabolism is not well understood. However,

Contemporary Questions and Answers

one study from New Zealand indicates that a significant loss in bone mineral density can be associated with the protracted use of Depo-Provera injections for birth control measures in otherwise normal women. Once these injections are discontinued, theoretically, the bone mineral density would slowly return to normal, but there is no real evidence to support this theory. Since you are approaching the age for the normal menopause, the long-term use of Depo-Provera injections may have reduced your bone mineral density enough to set you up for osteoporosis at an earlier age than even your mother. With this in mind, I would strongly suggest that you talk with your physician about scheduling a bone mineral density scan of both your spine and hips with the DEXA machine in the near future.

Question 3: Dr. Taylor, I had a total hysterectomy at age 28 due to endometriosis which did not respond to medical treatment. The surgeon told me that he also took my ovaries out. After the surgery, he sent me back to my gynecologist who did not recommend any sex steroid replacement. I am now 30 years old and married, but I do not enjoy sexual intercourse very much anymore. Sometimes sex just hurts. My husband complains about it and says that I have changed. I'm embarrassed to tell you that I don't have orgasms anymore like I used to. What can I do? I'm afraid that my husband will leave me if something is not done.

Answer: Your question is a very common one, but a sad one. Many physicians fail to prescribe the proper sex steroids after a total hysterectomy and ovaries removal in young women. It should be no surprise that the sex drive and sexual gratification are modulated by the sex steroids. Testosterone and anabolic-androgenic steroids are the body's own chemical aphrodisiacs as scientifically proven in the 1940s. Estrogenic steroids help to maintain the compliance of the vaginal mucosa, making it more spongy and soft. Also, estrogenic steroids play a major role in the formation and secretion of vaginal lubricants which are necessary for sexual pleasure. Since you have had your uterus removed, I would recommend a protocol which I have had good success with: (1) Estrace 0.5mg daily; (b) Winstrol 2mg daily for

Osteoporosis

calendar days 1–10 each month; (c) DEXA bone mineral density scan for your spine and hips; and (d) followup with your physician for symptoms or conditions which may arise and to tailor your sex steroid doses, if necessary.

Question 4: I am a 70-year-old white lady who went through the change of life about 25 years ago, and my doctor put me on a 2.5mg of Premarin daily back then for the hot flashes which I was experiencing. I had fewer hot flashes, but I retained fluid, had headaches and hypertension and gained weight. I told my doctor that I was still having some hot flashes and he increased my dose of Premarin and put me on a diuretic daily. My husband claimed that I was very moody then. Therefore, I decided to stop the Premarin on my own. Now, I have read in the newspaper about osteoporosis and I'm worried that I may have it. I have lost three inches of height. My physician told me years ago never to take estrogens again. What should I do?

Answer: You have a common dilemma with estrogenic steroid replacement which seems to be somewhat dose-related. Your problems may have also been related to the type of estrogenic steroids which you took many years ago. Unknowingly, your physician prescribed you an equine urine—derived conjugated estrogen at a relatively large dose to begin with and then an even larger dose when your symptoms did not resolve. This is a common mistake which some physicians have made and still make. Without the benefit of other information, I would make the following recommendations: (a) get a DEXA scan of both your spine and hips; (b) take 0.5mg of Estrace daily; (c) consider taking 2mg Winstrol daily for 10 days each month, especially if the DEXA scans indicate low or osteoporotic bone mineral densities; and (d) followup with your physician in order to tailor your sex steroid doses, if needed, to alleviate your symptoms and conditions.

Question 5: I am a 33-year-old white lady who is the wife of a chiropractor. I sustained a right hip fracture last year while I was playing tennis. I felt pain in my right groin area as I slid for a forehand shot; then I fell to the ground in pain. I really don't understand how this could have happened. I have been taking oral contraceptives for fifteen years and have had regular menstrual cycles. I have also taken regular injections of cortisone, about five or six times per year, for my allergies since I was twenty years old. I have had normal menstrual cycles since I was fourteen years old. I had a recent DEXA scan in your office which showed that I had a normal bone mineral density in my spine, but both of my hips had very severe osteoporosis. My hustand is an organic freak and he believes that natural herbs and vitamins will strengthen my hip bones along with physical therapy. What do you think?

Answer: There are many factors, known and perhaps unknown, which contribute to the condition of osteoporosis. One of the known factors is your regular injections of cortisone over the years for your allergies. Cortisone seems to bind to the androgen receptors on the osteoblast and inhibit normal bone formation and calcium incorporation into the bones. I have also seen several women who have taken oral contraceptives for years who have been tested with the DEXA scan and have normal bone mineral density in the spine and osteoporotic hips. My recommendations would be as follows: (a) discontinue the cortisone injections for your allergies. There are many other newer nonsteroidal medications which may help you. If they do not, then I would suggest allergy testing and desensitization techniques. (b) Make sure that you take at least 1500mg of elemental calcium supplements daily along with a multivitamin which gives you 600IU of vitamin D. (c) Take 2mg daily of Winstrol for the first 10 days of your menstrual cycle each month. And (d) have a repeat DEXA scan in six months to determine whether or not your bone mineral density is increasing.

Question 6: Dr. Taylor, I am a 36-year-old white woman who has had a hysterectomy three years ago for endometriosis. I have been treated with Danocrine for this condition since I was a teenager. I still have my ovaries, but I am worried that I might develop osteoporosis. I am currently on no medication at all. My mother and I now see eye-to-eye, but she used to be much taller than I was. My grandmother

Osteoporosis

just died in the hospital after she had a hip fracture. What do you suggest?

Answer: Danocrine is an anabolic-androgenic steroid and it is the sister of Winstrol. It has been known since the 1940s that anabolic-androgenic steroids are useful in the treatment of endometriosis. A few published studies have shown that Danocrine therapy *increases* bone mineral density in women with endometriosis. My suggestion would be to have a DEXA bone mineral density scan sometime within the next two years or so to see what your baseline levels are. Then, I would follow your physician's advice on how to proceed with your health care based on these findings.

Question 7: Dr. Taylor, I am an 81-year-old white woman with osteoporosis. I was referred for an DEXA test by my kidney doctor. I have never taken sex steroid replacement. I used to be an international concert organist in my youth. I still have my custom-made organ in my house, but for the last few years, I haven't been able to sit long enough to play it. My back, hands and fingers hurt when I attempt to play. I know I have osteoporosis and there is no hope. I use a walker to get around, but mostly I use a wheelchair. I live alone, for my husband died years ago. Can you help me play my organ again?

Answer: The medical studies from the 1940s suggest that there is no age which is too old to treat the pain and symptoms of osteoporosis with estrogen-androgen sex steroid therapy. Patients just seem to do much better overall. Of course, even the best therapy cannot reverse the damage which has already occurred, but it can be halted and the remaining bone structure can be strengthened. Also, anabolic-androgenic steroids help build muscle mass and strength, which is usually very important for elderly women. These steroids also enhance mood and decrease depression. Therefore, I would recommend that you begin my protocol of Estrace and Winstrol. I would also recommend a DEXA bone mineral density scan for a baseline study and the repeat studies every six months. [This patient, known to our clinic as "Old Claudia," followed my recommendations. Her initial bone density test indicated that she was very osteoporotic. She came in for her scheduled semiannual visits and rescans. Three years later, she appeared on our Christmas special TV program, "Bones, Hormones and Hot Flashes," but we videotaped her at home. At the age of 84 years, she played Christmas music on her organ for us on television. She no longer required a wheelchair or a walker to get around, for she walked on her own accord. She claimed that my therapy had made all of the difference.]

Question 8: I am a woman you have studied and I have osteoporosis. You prescribed Winstrol 2mg daily for 10 days each month as part of my treatment. My pharmacist told me that Winstrol is not indicated for osteoporosis. My primary care physician thinks that you are a "quack." What should I do?

Answer: Winstrol was indicated for the adjunct treatment of osteoporosis for decades, but in the early 1980s Winstrol was no longer approved for this therapy according to the FDA. Winstrol worked then and it works now. The factors behind the reasons why Winstrol is no longer approved by the FDA for the treatment of osteoporosis are covered within this book. Presently, there are a number of scientists researching the use of anabolic-androgenic steroids for osteoporosis therapy. The use of this sex steroid for this therapy is one which is renewed and it can be defended in any venue. My recommendations are to take Winstrol as prescribed and keep your follow-up appointments and DEXA scans.

Question 9: Dr. Taylor, I am a 60-year-old woman who is postmenopausal without symptoms. I live in a small town and there is no physician who specializes in osteoporosis care. I am healthy and I take no medications. My mother just recently had a hip fracture and now she can't walk. She is really going downhill. I am worried. My doctor, here, doesn't seem to really care that much about osteoporosis and I would like to know more about it. I seem to be shrinking in height like my mother did. What should I do?

Answer: A definitive osteoporosis scan and evaluation is truly available today for nearly everyone, even in small towns. Since the

Osteoporosis

follow-up appointment is usually only every six months or so, traveling a distance to receive the appropriate diagnosis and treatment is not that much of a hardship. I wouldn't hesitate to make an appointment for an evaluation and a DEXA scan this year.

Question 10: Dr. Taylor, I am a postmenopausal white women who doesn't believe in drugs. I take plenty of calcium every day. Isn't that good enough?

Answer: Chances are that taking calcium supplements alone for postmenopausal osteoporosis is not good enough. If it were, then why would I write a book about the need for sex steroid replacement therapy? Supplemental calcium is essential, but without the sex steroid stimulation of the osteoblast, the extra calcium is not incorporated into the bone and is lost through urination.

Question 11: I am a 63-year-old white woman who went through the menopause about 13 years ago. My doctor put me on Premarin 0.625mg daily and I have been taking it on a regular basis. I have gained about 25 pounds and I have a loss of sexual desire, which may be normal for my age. I am short, but lately I have had a difficult time seeing above my steering wheel. I have chronic neck and back pain. I take my calcium daily along with a multivitamin. I used to really enjoy sex with my husband, but now for years, I have really no interest; it has become more of a chore. My husband is a fit, attractive man who is always on me about my weight. I have been to several doctors with these complaints and I have not been satisfied with what I have been told. Are there any recommendations which you may have for me?

Answer: Your situation is not all that uncommon. Loss of sexual desire and loss of height are two major signs of sex steroid deficiency. In our clinic we have noted that about 50 percent of the women on Premarin alone eventually develop osteoporosis. Also, Premarin plays little, if any, role in sexual desire. Also, in many women, estrogen monotherapy can cause increased disposition of body fat. Therefore, my recommendations would include the following: (a) a DEXA bone mineral density scan within the year; (b) estrogen-androgen sex steroid replacement including Estrace 0.5mg daily and Winstrol 2mg daily for 10 days each month; and (c) follow-up visits with your physician for periodic reevaluation of your condition.

Question 12: Dr. Taylor, I am a white woman who was part of one of your initial studies on reversing osteoporosis. Over the past 18 months my bone mineral density has increased nearly 30 percent, which makes it normal again for my age. Should I continue the Estrace-Winstrol combination as before, or should I discontinue one or both of these sex steroids?

Answer: You are having no ill effects due to the Estrace-Winstrol therapy and I would lean towards continuing the prescribed protocol, unless adverse effects begin to surface. You have made a great deal of progress in a very short period of time. I know that you feel better about yourself from a self-esteem and body image point of view.

Question 13: I am a 57-year-old postmenopausal white woman who has been on Premarin since my menopause six years ago. A recent DEXA scan indicated that I had mild osteoporosis. My physician discontinued my Premarin therapy and started me on Fosamax. A few months later I began to experience pain during sexual intercourse with my husband. Can I begin taking my Premarin again?

Answer: Fosamax is a new nonhormonal drug for the treatment of osteoporosis in postmenopausal women. It is classified as a bisphosphonate which helps reduce bone resorption via osteoclast inhibition. The limited scientific studies indicate that Fosamax therapy can reverse bone mineral density losses at the rate of 2 to 4 percent per year. As far as the bone morphology changes seen, Fosamax therapy in rats and baboons indicates that the increased bone formation is normal. It may take further studies in humans to verify this point. In the clinical studies, a small number of postmenopausal women received estrogen while taking Fosamax with no adverse experiences attributed to the therapy. At this time, simultaneous use of sex steroid replacement and Fosamax to treat postmenopausal osteoporosis is not

Osteoporosis

recommended due to the lack of clinical experience. Therefore, I would advise that you discuss this situation with your physician, because you are not only experiencing osteoporosis, but other symptoms of lack of sex steroids.

Question 14: Dr. Taylor, I have heard that exercise is very important to prevent and treat postmenopausal osteoporosis. Can exercise actually cause fractures in patients who already have osteoporosis?

Answer: Various types of weight-bearing exercise seem to stimulate the osteoblast to some degree. But a woman's bones can become so fragile that even bending over to pick up a newspaper can cause the bones of the spine to fracture. In some cases, a woman with osteoporosis can fracture her hip just by bearing weight. In some of my severely osteoporotic women patients I have had to actually *restrict* them from exercise until we could achieve some reversal of their bone mineral density deficits.

Weight-bearing exercises are not the only useful forms of exercise that can prevent bone mineral density losses. There are some temporary changes which can result from prolonged continuous aerobic exercise which can result in bone mineral density enhancement. The adrenal gland is a gland which can be activated by stress, such as aerobic exercise, to excrete testosterone and other androgens. Also, aerobic exercise can cause a secretion of human growth hormone from the pituitary gland. Both androgens and growth hormone are osteoblast stimulators. Therefore, both strength training and aerobic training can be beneficial for maintaining strong bones and muscle tone.

Question 15: Dr. Taylor, I am a postmenopausal white woman who works out regularly. I have been studying whatever I can on the over-the-counter supplements for athletes sold in health food stores. I am currently taking supplemental boron and some of the literature which I have read indicates that it may strengthen bones. Can you comment on this?

Answer: Boron is a lightweight element on the periodic table. It is sold as a supplement in its trivalent form. To understand how boron may enhance bone mineral density, it is important to discuss some basic physiology of sex steroids. Most of the sex steroids in the body, once produced and secreted, are carried throughout the body by a spongelike molecule known as steroid hormone binding globulin. This globulin serves as a sort of reservoir for sex steroids. As it circulates in the bloodstream, this globulin releases tiny quantities of sex steroids to the appropriate tissues. Apparently, boron fills some of the holes in this spongelike globulin so that more of the sex steroid is released to the tissues. In this sense, boron's action may actually increase the active levels of sex steroids. There is little scientific evidence on the actual effects of boron on bone mineral density. It is certainly an area which needs further research.

Question 16: I am a postmenopausal white woman who has severe osteoporosis. My doctor has prescribed Calcimar for me and I have to go to his office thrice weekly for Calcimar injections. The injections are often painful and expensive. I had a QCT osteoporosis test three years ago, but I have had no retesting. The injections seem to help my neck and back pain temporarily. Recently, I stepped and missed the curb, fell and broke my hip. I use a walker now. Can you comment on Calcimar, and is there some other form of therapy which may help me now?

Answer: Calcimar is a form of calcitonin which is a hormone which inhibits the bone dissolving osteoclast. It has recently gained FDA approval for the treatment of osteoporosis. It is most beneficial in "high turnover" situations where patients have overactive osteoclasts. It will not stimulate new bone formation, however. Calcimar does seem to give temporary relief from pain, especially those which involve microfractures of the spine. It usually causes a 1 or 2 percent annual increase in bone mineral density over a two-year period, and then the bone material density effects seem to level off. The injections can be painful. Recently, a nasal spray form of calcitonin, Miacalcin, has been approved by the FDA for osteoporosis therapy. This form obviates the need for painful injections. Calcitonin drugs are recommended for women who refuse or cannot tolerate estrogens or in whom estrogens should not be used. There is major doubt, however, whether or not prolonged calcitonin drugs can reverse significant deficits in bone mineral density. And, of course, these drugs do not treat the other significant postmenopausal conditions.

Question 17: Dr. Taylor, I am a 59-year-old postmenopausal white woman who has been treated with Didronel for my osteoporosis. I had a QCT osteoporosis test to make the diagnosis, but I have not had any retesting over the past two years. I'm still having hot flashes, mood swings, vaginal dryness and no sexual desire. My doctor recommended that I take sex steroids; what do you think?

Answer: Didronel is a bisphosphonate drug which slows bone dissolving by inhibiting osteoclast function. It does not have FDA approval for treating osteoporosis. There was a major research study which looked at the effects of Didronel on postmenopausal osteoporosis; it showed that Didronel did have moderate effects on increasing bone mineral densities, but it seemed to produce *increases* in the incidence of bone fractures. Therefore the study was discontinued. Further studies are forthcoming. Of course, Didronel will not treat the other postmenopausal conditions which sex steroid replacement does. I would recommend that you take the time to discuss sex steroid replacement with your physician and have him schedule you for a DEXA scan for both your spine and hips. Combined use of sex steroids and Didronel is generally not recommended. Any combination of these drugs should be carefully considered based on an individual patient's circumstances.

Question 18: I have read in a magazine that fluoride therapy is the answer for the treatment of osteoporosis. I know that fluoride in the water can strengthen teeth; why not in bones?

Answer: Fluoride in the water has been shown to strengthen the *enamel* of teeth, not the jaw bone. Fluoride treatment does seem to produce a mild enhancement of bone mineral density, but it does so in a way that tends to produce abnormal bone structure. Therefore, fluoride increases bone mineral density to a small degree while causing weaker bone morphology and bone strength. Fluoride has not been approved by the FDA for the treatment of osteoporosis.

Question 19: I am a 70-year-old man with osteoporosis. My physician in Tennessee has me on a steroid therapy called Deca-Durabolin. I see him once a month for injections. He has a DEXA machine and I've shown good improvement with my osteoporosis over the past two years. I believe that Deca-Durabolin is an anabolic steroid. Can you comment on this therapy in men?

Answer: Deca-Durabolin is a long-acting injectable form of anabolic-androgenic steroid with a high therapeutic index. It has been shown to stimulate osteoblast activity and cause normal bone structure. Men who have osteoporosis should not take anabolic-androgenic steroids if they have prostate cancer, which is common in elderly men. Before I could recommend this type of sex steroid therapy for osteoporosis in men, I would have to rule out, as completely as possible, prostatic cancer. I don't believe that anabolic-androgenic steroids cause prostate cancer, but these steroids can make prostate cancer grow and spread faster. I would have to perform a digital prostate examination and order a prostate cancer blood test known as prostate specific antigen (PSA) prior to prescribing this therapy. I have discussed the use of long-acting anabolic-androgenic steroid replacement for osteoporosis therapy in men with a few researchers. It seems that after a year or two there is some plateauing of effects with the long-acting steroids. I believe that there may be some tolerance in these steroids given in this fashion. Therefore, I still prefer a protocol that calls for cyclical use of shorter acting anabolic-androgenic steroids in both women and men.

Discussion

Finding the right physician to discuss some of the more intimate details about postmenopausal issues may prove to be difficult. Learning about these postmenopausal issues takes time to understand, and usually not all of these issues can be covered within the setting of a single office visit. Physicians vary in their willingness and ability to teach. My recommendation on physician choice is to find one with whom you can share very intimate details about your life without fear that the physician's attitude will be judgmental.

There are many questions which I have not been able to address regarding menopause and osteoporosis. Treatment during the menopause and postmenopausal years may involve several types of physicians, and there is a real need for these various types of physicians to reach agreement about the therapy of postmenopausal osteoporosis. Today physicians in nearly every specialty tend to have their own slant on this issue.

Afterword

The sex steroids produced by the human body play a variety of roles in our lives. By denying that these powerful sex steroid molecules affect our physical and mental well-being, we bury our heads in the sand like an ostrich, and as the pages of this text have shown, that is precisely the approach that the medical profession has taken. The result has been the osteoporosis epidemic. Gaining a better understanding of these sex steroids can be a valuable contribution to one's maturing process as a human being.

When we consider the factors which limit human longevity, there is no biological reason for the skeleton to be among them. But longevity will be curtained for thousands and thousands of women with osteoporosis this year. It is my hope that this book will influence enough patients and physicians to control the osteoporosis epidemic.

Bibliography

Albright, F., E. Bloomberg, and P. H. Smith. "Postmenopausal Osteoporosis." *Trans. Assoc. Am. Phys.* 1940; 55:1940.

____, P. H. Smith, and A. M. Richardson. "Postmenopausal Osteoporosis: Its Clinical Features." *Journal of the American Medical Association.* 1941; 116:2465.

Aloia, K. F., A. Kapoor, and A. Vaswani. "Changes in Body Composition Following Therapy of Osteoporosis with Methandrostenolone." *Metabolism* 1981:1076.

Benton, M.N. C., A.J. P. Yates, and S. Rogers. "Stanozolol Stimulates Remodeling of Trabecular Bone and Net Formation of Bone at the Endocordial Surface." *Clinical Science.* 1991; 81:543.

Berubger, T.R.O., J. Ardill, and H.M.A. Taggart. "Effects of Calcium and Stanozolol on Calcitonin Secretion in Patients with Femoral Neck Fracture." *Bone Min.* 1986; 1:289.

Brown-Sequard, C. E. "Experience Démontrant la Puissance Dynamogenique Chez l'Homme d'un Liquide Extrait de Testicules d'Animaux." *Arch. de Physiol.* 1889; 1:651.

Butendant, A., and G. Hanish. "Uber Testosteron, Umwandlund des Dehydro-androsterons in Androstendiol aus Cholesterin." *Ztschr. f. Physiol. Chem.* 1935; 237:89.

Callantine, M. R., P. L. Martin, and O. T. "Bolding: Micronized 17-beta

Bibliography

Estradiol for Oral Estrogen Therapy in Menopausal Women." *Obstet. Gynecol.* 1975; 46(1):37.

Chestnut, C. H., W. B. Nelp, and D. J. Baylink. "Effect of Methandrostenolone on Postmenopausal Wasting as Assessed by Changes in Total Bone Mineral Mass." *Metabolism* 1977; 26:267.

———, J. L. Ivey, and H. E. Gruber. "Stanozolol in Postmenopausal Osteoporosis: Therapeutic Efficacy and Possible Mechanisms of Action." *Metabolism* 1983; 32:571.

Couch, M., R. E. Preston, and R. G. Malia. "Changes in Plasma Osteocalcin Concentrations Following Treatment with Stanozolol." *Clinical Chim. Acta* 1986; 158:43.

de Kruif, P. *The Male Hormone.* New York: Harcourt, Brace and Company, 1945.

Ettinger, B., H. K. Genant, and P. Steiger. "Low-dose Micronized 17-beta Estradiol Prevents Bone Loss in Postmenopausal Women." *American Journal Obstetrics/Gynecology.* 1992; 166(2):479.

Fruehan, A. E., and T. F. Frawley. "Current Status of Anabolic Steroids." *Journal of the American Medical Association.* 1963; 184(7):527.

Gennari, C., D. AgnusDei, and S. Gonnelli. "Effects of Nandrolone Decanoate Therapy on Bone Mass and Calcium Metabolism in Women with Established Postmenopausal Osteoporosis: A Double Blind Placebo-Controlled Study." *Maturitas* 1989; 11:187.

Greenblatt, R. B. Androgenic Therapy in Women. *Journal of Clinical Endocrinology* 1942; 2:65.

———. "The Use of Androgens in the Menopause and Other Gynecic Disorders." *Obstetrics Gynecol. N. America* 1987; 14(1):251.

Harrison, T. R. *Harrison's Principles of Internal Medicine.* New York: McGraw-Hill, 1977.

Hassager, C., L. T. Jensen, and J. S. Johansen. "The Carboxy-Terminal Propeptide of Type I Procollagen in Serum as a Marker of Bone Formation: The Effect of Nandrolone Decanoate and Female Sex Hormones." *Metabolism* 1991; 40:205.

———, ———, and J. Podenphant. "Collagen Synthesis in Postmenopausal Women During Therapy with Anabolic Steroid or Female Sex Hormones." *Metabolism* 1990; 39:1167.

———, B. L. Riis, and J. Podenphant. "Nandrolone Deconate Treatment of Postmenopausal Osteoporosis for 2 Years and Effects of Withdrawal." *Maturitas* 1989; 11:305.

Bibliography

Henneman, P. H., and S. Wallach. "The Use of Androgens and Estrogens and Their Metabolic Effects: A Review of the Prolonged Use of Estrogens and Androgens in Postmenopausal and Senile Osteoporosis." *Arch. Intern. Med.* 1957; 100:715.

Johansen, J., C. Hassager, and J. Podenphant. "Treatment of Postmenopausal Osteoporosis: Is the Anabolic Steroid Nandrolone Decanoate a Candidate?" *Bone Min.* 1989; 6:77.

Judd, H. C., G. E. Judd, and W. E. Lucas. "Endocrine Function of the Postmenopausal Ovary: Concentration of Androgens and Estrogens in Ovaries and Peripheral Vein Blood. *J. Clin. Endocrinol. Metab.* 1974; 39:1020.

Longcope, C. "Adrenal and Gonadal Androgenic Secretion in Normal Females." *J. Clin. Endocrinol. Metab.* 1986; 15:213.

Mikhail, G. "Sex Steroids in the Blood." *Clin. Obstet. Gynecol.* 1967; 10:29.

Need, A. G., H. A. Morris, and T. F. Hartley. "Effects of Nandrolone Decanoate on Forearm Mineral Density and Calcium Metabolism in Osteoporotic Postmenopausal Women." *Calif. Tissue Int.* 1987; 41:7.

Ray, O. *Drugs, Society and Human Behavior.* St. Louis: C. V. Mosby Company, 1978.

Reifenstein, E. C. "The Relationship of Steroid Hormones to the Development and Management of Osteoporosis in Aging People." *Clin. Ortho. Rel. Res.* 1957; 10:207.

_____ and F. Albright. "Metabolic Effects of Steroid Hormones in Osteoporosis." *J. Clin. Invest.* 1947; 26:24.

Riggs, B. L., J. Jowsey, and R. S. Goldsmith. "Short and Long-Term Effects of Estrogen and Synthetic Anabolic Hormones in Postmenopausal Osteoporosis." *J. Clin. Invest.* 1972; 51:1659.

Ruzicka, L., A. Wettstein, and H. Kaegi. "Sexual Hormone VIII Darstellung von Testosteron Unter Anweducng Gemischeter Ester." *Helv. Chim. Acta* 1935; 18:1487.

Salmon, U. J., and S. H. Geist. "Effects of Androgens Upon Libido in Women." *J. Clin. Endocrinol. Metab.* 1943; 3:235.

Sherwin, B. B., and M. M. Gelfand. "Differential Symptoms Response to Parenteral Estrogen and/or Androgen Administration in the Surgical Menopause." *Am. J. Obstet. Gynecol.* 1985; 151:153.

_____ and _____. "Effects of Parenteral Administration of Estrogen and Androgen on Plasma Hormone Levels and Hot Flashes in the Surgical Menopause." *Am. J. Obstet. Gynecol.* 1984; 148:552.

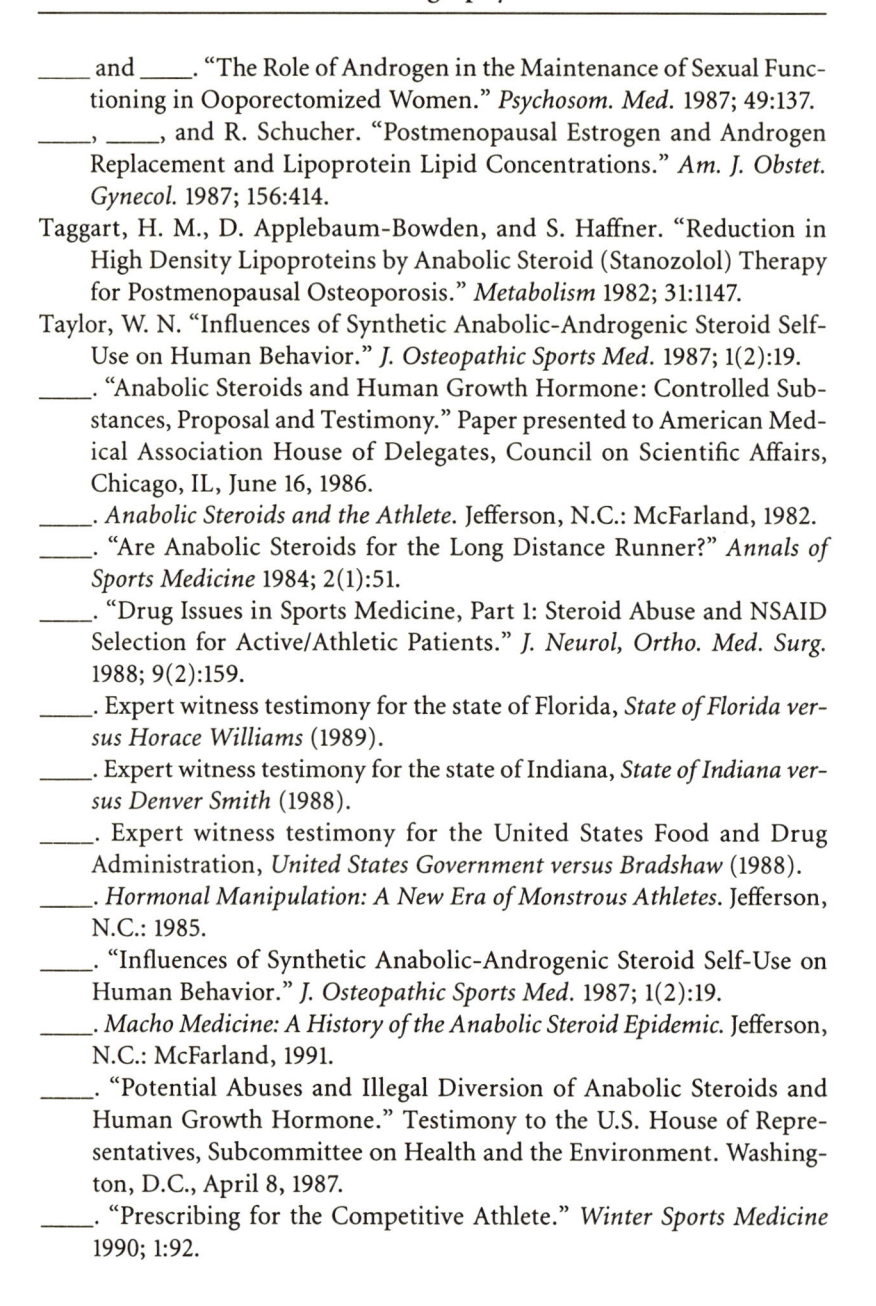

_____ and _____. "The Role of Androgen in the Maintenance of Sexual Functioning in Ooporectomized Women." *Psychosom. Med.* 1987; 49:137.

_____, _____, and R. Schucher. "Postmenopausal Estrogen and Androgen Replacement and Lipoprotein Lipid Concentrations." *Am. J. Obstet. Gynecol.* 1987; 156:414.

Taggart, H. M., D. Applebaum-Bowden, and S. Haffner. "Reduction in High Density Lipoproteins by Anabolic Steroid (Stanozolol) Therapy for Postmenopausal Osteoporosis." *Metabolism* 1982; 31:1147.

Taylor, W. N. "Influences of Synthetic Anabolic-Androgenic Steroid Self-Use on Human Behavior." *J. Osteopathic Sports Med.* 1987; 1(2):19.

_____. "Anabolic Steroids and Human Growth Hormone: Controlled Substances, Proposal and Testimony." Paper presented to American Medical Association House of Delegates, Council on Scientific Affairs, Chicago, IL, June 16, 1986.

_____. *Anabolic Steroids and the Athlete.* Jefferson, N.C.: McFarland, 1982.

_____. "Are Anabolic Steroids for the Long Distance Runner?" *Annals of Sports Medicine* 1984; 2(1):51.

_____. "Drug Issues in Sports Medicine, Part 1: Steroid Abuse and NSAID Selection for Active/Athletic Patients." *J. Neurol, Ortho. Med. Surg.* 1988; 9(2):159.

_____. Expert witness testimony for the state of Florida, *State of Florida versus Horace Williams* (1989).

_____. Expert witness testimony for the state of Indiana, *State of Indiana versus Denver Smith* (1988).

_____. Expert witness testimony for the United States Food and Drug Administration, *United States Government versus Bradshaw* (1988).

_____. *Hormonal Manipulation: A New Era of Monstrous Athletes.* Jefferson, N.C.: 1985.

_____. "Influences of Synthetic Anabolic-Androgenic Steroid Self-Use on Human Behavior." *J. Osteopathic Sports Med.* 1987; 1(2):19.

_____. *Macho Medicine: A History of the Anabolic Steroid Epidemic.* Jefferson, N.C.: McFarland, 1991.

_____. "Potential Abuses and Illegal Diversion of Anabolic Steroids and Human Growth Hormone." Testimony to the U.S. House of Representatives, Subcommittee on Health and the Environment. Washington, D.C., April 8, 1987.

_____. "Prescribing for the Competitive Athlete." *Winter Sports Medicine* 1990; 1:92.

Bibliography

———. "Prescribing for the Competitive Athlete: Part 1." *J. Osteopathic Sports Med.* 1988; 2(1):12.

———. "Prescribing for the Competitive Athlete: Part 2." *J. Osteopathic Sports Med.* 1988; 2(2):16.

———. "Super Athletes Made to Order?" *Psychology Today* 1985; 19(5):66.

———. "Synthetic Anabolic-Androgenic Steroids: A Plea for Controlled Substance Status." *Physician and Sports Medicine* 1987; 15:140.

——— and C. Alanis. "Triple Sex Steroid Replacement Therapy for Osteoporosis After Surgical Menopause." *N. Neurol. Ortho. Med. Surg.* 1992; 13:16.

———, ———, and D. J. Wigley. "Oral Cyclical Stanozolol and Daily Micronized 17-beta Estradiol Combination Therapy for Postmenopausal Osteoporosis: A Preliminary Report." *J. Neurol. Orthop. Med. Surg.* 1994, 15:25.

——— and A. B. Black. "Pervasive Anabolic Steroid Use Among Health Club Athletes." *Annals of Sports Medicine* 1987; 3:3.

Tostenson, A. N. A., D. I. Rosenthal, and L. J. Melton. "Cost Effectiveness of Screening Perimenopausal White Women for Osteoporosis: Bone Densitometry and Hormone Replacement Therapy." *Ann. Int. Med.* 1990; 113:594.

Vaishnav, R., J. N. Beresford, and J. A. Gallagher. "Effects of the Anabolic Steroid Stanozolol on Cells Derived from Human Bone." *Clin. Sci.* 1988; 74:455.

Yates, A. J. P., R. E. S. Gray, and R. C. Percival. "Skeletal Effects of Stanozolol in Osteoporosis." In C. Christiansen, C. D. Arnaud and B. E. C. Nordin, eds., *Osteoporosis I. Proceedings of Copenhagen International Symposium on Osteoporosis, 1984*; 509.

About the Author

William N. Taylor, MD, is the author of three highly regarded books on drug abuse in athletics and one on marathon running. He graduated from the University of West Florida in 1975 with a bachelor of science degree in chemistry, earned his master of science degree in chemical and polymer engineering from the University of Tennessee in 1976, and, after working in the plastics industry, earned his doctor of medicine degree from the University of Miami School of Medicine in 1981. He completed his PGY−1 year in residency at the Pensacola Educational Program in 1982.

Dr. Taylor has served as an expert in a number of positions, including the American College of Sports Medicine, which awarded him the status of Fellow in 1985; the United States Olympic Drug Control Program, in which he participated from 1984 to 1988; and the American Academy of Sports Physicians, where he served on the Board of Governors in 1986. In 1988 he served as an expert witness for the United States Food and Drug Administration.

Dr. Taylor is a respected lecturer who spent nearly four years delivering his lectures on "Drug Issues in Sports Medicine" to major league baseball, to the California Drug Enforcement Agency, and to

About the Author

physician and drug counseling groups nationwide. He has appeared in several television documentaries on anabolic-androgenic steroid abuse and human growth hormone abuse. He has been widely published in the scientific press and was responsible for spearheading the movement to have anabolic-androgenic steroids placed on the controlled substance list by an act of Congress in 1991.

Dr. Taylor had the first dual-energy X-ray densitometer (DEXA) in the state of Florida in 1990 and has focused much of his time since then in the field of osteoporosis. He has published two scientific articles which showed that the proper use of sex steroids can reverse and perhaps cure osteoporosis in women. As of 1996 he is an associate professor in the Department of Exceptional and Physical Education at the University of Central Florida in Orlando.

Index

acne 26
addiction, drug 22
adherence to therapy 59, 60
adrenal glands 50, 88
aerobic capacity 33
AIDS 9
amenorrhea 65
American Medical Association 30, 54
anabolic-androgenic steroids (androgens) vii, 15, 20, 21, 23, 24, 25, 28, 29, 30, 31, 32, 33, 34, 35, 39, 44, 45, 49, 51, 56, 57, 58, 59, 60, 61, 62, 63, 64, 65, 71, 75–77; anabolic functions of 33, 34; androenic functions of 34; therapeutic index of 34, 35, 91
Anabolic Steroids and the Athlete 24, 34
Anadrol 34
"andropause" 20, 50, 80
anemia 29
angina pectoris 29
antigonadotropic steroid 77
anxiety neurosis 36

aphrodisiacs 24
aspirin 64
athletic performance 29, 30, 77

bawdy overtones 27
bed wetting 29
Berlind, Dr. Melvyn 26
birth control pills 39, 79, 80
bisphosphonates 49, 57, 62, 90
blood clots 39
Board of Medicine 70
body fat 33, 39
bodybuilders, female 65
bone fractures 1, 49, 63
bone metabolism 26, 48, 49, 50
bone mineral density 5, 16, 19, 20, 32, 33, 34, 35, 39, 43, 51, 52, 56, 60, 61, 62, 72, 80
bone resorption 27, 48, 49
Bones, Hormones and Hot Flashes 70, 85
boron 88, 89

Index

breasts: cancer of 2, 37, 39; swelling of 39; tenderness of 39

Calcimar 57, 89
calcitonin 49, 57, 89
calcium supplementation 15, 43, 55, 56, 67, 83, 86
cancer: breast 2, 37, 39; ovarian 2
cardiologists 73, 74
chiropractic physicians 16, 52, 82
cholesterol levels 59, 62
Ciba 34
clitoral enlargement 65
coffee 64
conjugated estrogens 36–37, 82
controlled substances 71
cortisone 83
credibility, loss of 40

Danocrine 77, 83, 84
Deca-Durabolin 34, 57, 91
delayed puberty 29
dental physicians 52, 77
Depo-Provera 80, 81
Depo-Testosterone 34, 57
depression 29, 35, 36, 38, 59, 67
diabetes 52
Dianabol 34, 57, 65, 90
"dowager's hump" 7
Drug Enforcement Agency 22
dual-energy X-ray absorptiometer (DEXA) 52, 53, 54, 55, 61, 62, 64, 70, 72, 74, 75, 76, 80, 81, 82, 84, 86, 87, 90, 91

electrolyte retention 34
elixirs 22
"empty nest syndrome" 36
endometriosis 29, 83, 84

endurance 33
energy level 59, 60, 62, 67, 79
"entrepreneurs" 55
enuresis 29
epidemic, osteoporosis 1, 8, 10, 19, 28, 41, 43
equine-derived conjugated estrogens 36–37, 82
Estrace 38, 39, 57, 62, 63, 81, 82, 84
Estratest 57, 71
estrogen/androgen combination therapy vii, 28, 33, 44, 56, 57, 58, 59, 60, 61, 62, 63, 70, 71, 72, 75, 76, 81, 87
estrogenic steroids (estrogens) vii, 15, 20, 21, 26, 27, 33, 35, 36, 37, 38, 39, 40, 43, 44, 45, 48, 49, 50, 51, 56, 57, 58, 59, 60, 62, 72, 81, 90; adverse effects of 39
ethanol 22, 64

facial hair 26, 34, 65
FDA 11, 22, 28, 31, 32, 52, 56, 65, 85
fluid retention 39, 82
fluoride 49, 90, 91
fluoroxymesterone 34
"forgotten" sex steroids 44
Fosamax 57, 87, 88
Freud, Dr. Sigmund 27
fungi 22

Gambrell, Dr. 20
generic drugs 31
Gestapo 30
Goldman, Alex Dr. 25
grand rounds 76
Greenblatt, Robert B., M.D. vii, viii, 20, 25, 57
growth factors 49
growth hormone 49, 88

104

Index

growth stimulator 29
gynecologists 70, 71, 72, 76, 77, 80, 81

hallucinogens 22
Halotestin 34
Hamilton, Alexander 11
Harrison's Principles of Internal Medicine 27, 28, 35, 36, 44, 65
health food stores 72, 88
health insurance 7
heart disease 2, 59, 60, 74
height loss 3, 16, 82, 83, 84, 86
herbs 22, 72
hip fractures 1, 2, 7, 32, 45, 53, 71, 75, 82
Hitler, Adolf 30
hospital politics 55
hot flashes 38, 59, 67, 82, 90
hucksters 28
hyperlipidemia 29
hypertension 29, 39, 82
hypochrondriasis 36
hypothyroidism 52
hysterectomy 67, 81, 83
hysteria 36, 67

ibuprofen 64
immune system depression 29
impotence 29
insulin 26, 52

Johnson, Ben 63

kidney stones 43

libido 26, 27, 34, 59, 60, 62, 65, 67, 73, 80, 86, 90

"little old lady" 9
longevity 33, 59

Macho Medicine: A History of the Anabolic Steroid Epidemic 24
male menopause 29
manipulation, spinal 16
marijuana 22
masculinization 28, 44, 58, 63
"medical authorities" 10, 19, 21, 22, 40, 43, 44, 45, 66
"medical dynamite" 24
medical politics 29, 31, 37, 66
Medicare 8, 54, 74
melatonin 49
memory loss 59
menopause: definition of 20; symptoms of 29, 36, 58
"menopause syndrome" 35, 36
methandrostenolone 34, 65
Miacalcin 57, 89
microfactures 16
mood swings 39, 67, 90
muscle mass 28, 33, 64, 65
myleofibrosis 29

nandrolone decanoate 34
NASA 66
National Academy of Sciences 65
National Osteoporosis Foundation 1
Nazi experimentation 30
neurosurgeon 74
night sweats 67
nitrogen retention 34
Nobel Prize 23
Nolvadex 49
nursing home 45

obesity 36
obsessive-compulsive illness 36

105

Index

Ogen 57
Olympic Games 30, 63
oocytes 51
opium 22
oral contraceptives 39, 80, 83
Organon 34
orgasmic response 26
osteoblast stimulator 32, 33, 34, 35, 43, 49, 50, 56, 57, 62, 63, 64, 65, 88
osteoblasts 21, 35, 36, 48, 50, 51, 52, 55, 56, 57, 58, 59, 60–65
osteoclasts 21, 35, 36, 48, 49, 50, 51, 52, 56, 58, 59, 89
osteopathic physicians 52
osteopenia 6
osteoporosis: cure for 5, 32, 41, 64; definition of 5; diagnosis of 52, 53, 54, 55; FDA-approved drugs for 31, 32, 56, 57, 65, 66; financial costs of 1, 8, 41, 53; myths about 15; national screening for 6, 32; nomenclature mistakes concerning 23, 27; reversal of 15, 24, 32, 33, 47; risks of 6
ovarian cancer 2
ovarian involution 20, 38, 60
ovarian "sputtering" 20, 80
oxymesterone 34

package inserts: Dianabol 65; Winstrol 31, 65
parathyroid hormone 49
perimenopause 20, 36, 38, 50, 51, 52, 53, 58, 80
personality changes 39
peyote 22
pharmaceutical industry 22, 31, 36
pharmacists 85
phobic states 36
Physician's Desk Reference 31, 65, 66
podiatric physicians 52, 76

political stances 10, 26
polypeptide hormones 48, 49
poppy 22
Premarin 36, 37, 38, 39, 52, 57, 62, 71, 72, 86, 87
premature babies 29
premenstrual condition 79
prescription writing, habitual 37
Prevention magazine 20
preventive medicine 7, 40
Procrustes 45
progesterogenic steroids (progesterones) 20, 51, 61, 62, 63, 80, 81
prostate specific antigen (PSA) 91
Provera 62
"psych cases" 36
psychiatrists 16, 27, 36, 52, 58, 67
psychologists 16, 27, 36, 67
psychotic illness 29
pubic hair 34

qualitative computer tomography (QCT) 54, 55, 74, 75, 89, 90
quality of life 33, 59, 60
quantity of life 33, 59, 60

Raynaud's syndrome 29
Redmond, Dr. Geoffrey 30
rheumatoid arthritis 29, 73
rheumatologist 72, 73

Searle 34
sex drive 26, 27, 34, 59, 60, 62, 65, 67, 73, 79, 80, 86, 90
sex steroids vii, 2, 5, 6, 15, 19, 23, 24, 27, 30, 32, 33, 36, 37, 38, 39, 44, 45, 47, 48, 49, 52, 53, 58–68, 73, 78; byproducts of 37; "gender specificity" of 25, 26

Index

sexual attractiveness 36
sexual behavior 57, 64
sexual intercourse 67, 81
sexual pleasure 26, 81, 86
"sexual TNT" 24
Sheehy, Gail 17
silent killer 8
"small bladder syndrome" 68
societal apathy 3
space travel 66
sports medicine 30, 64
"standard of care" 48, 53
stanozolol 31, 32, 33, 34, 57, 62, 63, 64, 65, 66, 71, 83, 84, 85
strokes 39
stromal cells 80
suntanning 29
surgical physicians 52

tamoxifen 49
tax burden 8
Technology Assessment Group 54
testosterone 15, 23, 24, 25, 26, 27, 28, 29, 30, 31, 34, 35, 39, 44, 50, 81
therapeutic index 34, 35, 91
thrombophlebitis 39
thyroid hormone 52
tooth loss 77, 78

ungratified sexuality 36
United States Congress 31, 70
United States Olympic Committee's Drug Control Program 77
Upjohn 34
urinary bladder 68
urinary incontinence 68
urine, equine 36–37, 82
uterine cancer 2, 37, 61

vaginal compliance 59
vaginal mucosa 67
vaginal secretions 59, 81, 90
vitamin D 49, 83
voice changes 26, 34, 65

weight bearing exercise 49
Wells, H.G. 13
Winstrol 31, 32, 33, 34, 57, 62, 63, 64, 65, 66, 71, 76, 77, 83, 84, 85
Winthrop Pharmaceutic Co. 31, 34, 77
women's groups 10
wrinkling 59

X-rays 16, 54, 55, 77